RNCM

The Comprehensive Guide for the

Hospice Nurse Case Manager

For Alan

Table of Contents

Chapter 6: The Death Visit

- Pronouncing the death of a hospice patient
- Preparing the body of the deceased
- Steps to take after death has occurred

Chapter 7: Documentation and Legal Issues

- Importance of accurate and thorough documentation
- Understanding legal and ethical considerations in hospice care
- Maintaining confidentiality and HIPAA compliance

Chapter 8: Working with Special Populations

- Providing hospice care to older adults
- Caring for terminally ill children and their families
- Supporting patients with advanced dementia and other cognitive impairments

Chapter 9: Advanced Care Planning

- Discussing end-of-life wishes with patients and their families
- Making decisions about life-sustaining treatments
- Advanced Directives and Power of Attorney

Chapter 10: The Importance of Hospice Care and the Role of the Case Manager

- The positive impact of hospice care on patients and their families
- The importance of the hospice case manager in providing high-quality care
- The rewards and challenges of being a hospice case manager

Chapter 1

Introduction to Hospice Care

As someone who has dedicated their nursing career to the compassionate care of seniors and those nearing the end of life, I understand the unique challenges and rewards that come with this demanding but deeply fulfilling work. I decided to write this book to serve as a source of support, inspiration, and practical guidance for those of us who have chosen to walk alongside our patients and their families during some of the most difficult and meaningful moments of their lives.

During my experience in hospice care, I learned firsthand the importance of maintaining a compassionate and supportive presence for those who are facing terminal illnesses. I am grateful for the opportunity to share my knowledge and experience with you, and I hope that this book will serve as a valuable resource as we continue to walk with our patients on their end-of-life journey.

Hospice care is specialized medical care provided to individuals with a terminal illness who are no longer seeking curative treatment. Instead, it is focused on providing comfort, support, and symptom management to patients and their families, and aims to improve their quality of life during the end-of-life stage. Hospice care can be provided in a variety of settings, including the patient's home, a hospice facility, or a nursing home. The interdisciplinary hospice team typically includes doctors, nurses, social workers, chaplains, and trained volunteers, who work together to provide comprehensive care to patients and their families.

In addition to medical care, hospice also offers emotional and spiritual support to patients and their loved ones, helping them cope with terminal illness and end-of-life challenges. Hospice care is a holistic approach that recognizes the importance of addressing the physical, emotional, social, and spiritual needs of patients and their families. It is an alternative to aggressive medical treatment that may not provide additional benefit to the patient and instead focuses on providing comfort and quality of life.

When caring for patients who are nearing the end of their life, the focus shifts to maintaining and improving their quality of life as much as possible. This means addressing not only their physical needs, but also their emotional, social, and spiritual needs.

One of the keys to focusing on quality of life is to listen to the patient's concerns and preferences. Each person is unique and has their own individual priorities and values. By taking the time to understand what matters most to the patient, we can help them live their remaining time in a way that is meaningful and fulfilling to them.

Providing comfort measures to alleviate pain and other symptoms are an essential component to effective hospice care. This can help the patient feel more comfortable and at ease, which can significantly improve their overall quality of life.

Ultimately, the goal of focusing on a patient's quality of life is to enable them to live as fully as possible in the time they have remaining, and to help them experience a sense of peace and dignity as they approach the end of their life.

The *National Hospice and Palliative Care Organization (NHPCO)* is a leading advocacy and education organization that promotes and supports hospice and palliative care. According to the NHPCO, hospice care is a model of care that focuses on providing comfort, support, and symptom management to individuals with a terminal illness and their families. It is an interdisciplinary approach that includes a team of professionals who work together to provide comprehensive care.

According to the National Hospice and Palliative Care Organization, hospice care "provides comprehensive medical, emotional, and spiritual care for individuals with a terminal illness and their families, emphasizing quality of life." The NHPCO emphasizes that hospice care is about more than just medical treatment, but also includes emotional and spiritual support for patients and their loved ones. The NHPCO is dedicated to improving the quality of hospice and palliative care through education, research, and advocacy.

The term "*hospice*" originated in medieval Europe, where it referred to a place of shelter and care for travelers and the sick. However, the history of hospice care dates back to ancient times when people who were dying were often cared for by their families or religious communities. In the Middle Ages, hospices were established as places where travelers and the sick could receive food, shelter, and medical care. These early hospices were often associated with religious institutions and were run by volunteers who provided care and support to those in need.

In the 19th and 20th centuries, the concept of hospice care began to evolve. However, it was not until the 1960s that the modern hospice movement began to take shape. In the United Kingdom, Dr. Cicely Saunders established the first modern hospice in 1967, called St. Christopher's Hospice. She believed dying patients should be treated with compassion and dignity and focused on providing palliative care to manage their symptoms and improve their quality of life. Dr. Saunders was a pioneer in hospice care, and her work inspired the development of hospice programs in other countries, including the United States.

For further reading: Cicely Saunders: A Life and Legacy by David Clark provides a fascinating biography of this remarkable woman and healthcare professional.

Dr. Elisabeth Kubler-Ross was a Swiss-American psychiatrist and author who is well known for her work in the field of hospice care and end-of-life issues. In the 1960s, Dr. Kubler-Ross began working as a psychiatrist at the University of Chicago, where she encountered many terminally ill patients and became interested in the psychological and emotional aspects of death and dying.

In 1969, she published her groundbreaking book, *"On Death and Dying,"* which outlined the five stages of grief that many people experience when faced with the loss of a loved one: denial, anger, bargaining, depression, and acceptance. She also became a leading advocate for the rights of the dying and for the importance of providing compassionate and supportive care to patients in the end-of-life phase.

Throughout her career, Dr. Kubler-Ross wrote numerous books and articles on end-of-life care and grief, and she lectured extensively on these topics around the world. She received many awards and honors for her work, including the Presidential Medal of Freedom in 1969. Her work has had a lasting impact on the way that hospice care is provided and has helped to improve the quality of life for countless patients and their families.

Florence Wald was an American nurse and healthcare administrator who is well known for her contributions to the development of hospice care. She was born on April 19, 1917, in New Haven, Connecticut, and received her nursing degree from Mount Holyoke College in 1939.

In the 1960s, Wald began working as a nursing administrator at Yale-New Haven Hospital, where she became interested in the care of terminally ill patients. She became particularly concerned with the lack of support and comfort available to these patients and their families, and she began to explore ways to improve the end-of-life experience.

In the late 1960s, Wald began working with Dr. Elisabeth Kubler-Ross. Together, they developed the concept of modern hospice care, which focused on providing specialized support and comfort to terminally ill patients and their families.

In 1974, Wald helped to establish the first hospice program in the United States, which was located at Yale-New Haven Hospital. She served as the director of this program for many years and was instrumental in its success.

Throughout her career, Wald worked tirelessly to promote the concept of hospice care and to improve the end-of-life experience for patients and their families. She received many awards and honors for her work, including the Presidential Medal of Freedom in 1999. Wald passed away on November 8, 2008, but her legacy in the field of hospice care lives on.

The New Haven Hospice program established by Wald was the first of its kind in the country and was designed to provide care and support to terminally ill patients and their families. The program was established in response to a growing need for specialized care for terminally ill patients, who often suffered from chronic pain, mental and emotional distress, and other symptoms associated with their illnesses.

The volunteers who established the hospice program in New Haven were motivated to provide compassionate and dignified care to terminally ill patients and their families. They believed that patients should be able to receive care and support in the comfort of their own homes, rather than in a hospital or other institutional setting. As such, the program focused on providing home-based care and support to terminally ill patients and their families, including medical care, emotional support, and practical assistance with activities of daily living.

In the decades that followed, the hospice program in New Haven grew and evolved, and similar programs began to be established in other parts of the country. Today, hospice care is an integral part of the healthcare system in the United States. It is provided by a wide range of organizations, including hospitals, home health agencies, and nonprofit organizations. As a result, hospice care is now considered a valuable and vital aspect of end-of-life care and is widely recognized for its ability to provide patients and their families with high-quality, compassionate care.

In the United States, the *Medicare Hospice Benefit* was established in 1982, providing financial support for hospice programs. This marked a significant milestone in developing hospice care, as it allowed more patients to access this specialized medical care. In modern times, hospice care is offered by a wide range of organizations, including nonprofit hospices, for-profit hospices, and hospital-based hospices. It is an integral part of the healthcare system, providing compassionate and supportive care to individuals facing the end of life.

The Hospice Medicare benefit is a program that provides financial support for hospice care for patients with terminal illnesses. The goal of the Hospice Medicare benefit is to help patients and their families manage their symptoms, improve their quality of life, and provide emotional and spiritual support during the end-of-life process.

When patients elect to use the Hospice Medicare benefit, they are entitled to a comprehensive package of services, including medical care, pain management, symptom control, and emotional and spiritual support. The Hospice Medicare benefit covers these services for the patient and their family, and the cost of medications, medical equipment, and other supplies related to the patient's hospice care.

The Hospice Medicare benefit has several advantages. For example, it provides financial support for hospice care, which can be expensive and may not be covered by other forms of insurance. It also provides access to a team of healthcare professionals specializing in hospice care, which can be helpful for patients and their families dealing with a terminal illness.

However, the Hospice Medicare benefit also has some disadvantages. For example, it requires that the patient have a terminal illness, which means they must be expected to live for six months or less to qualify for the benefit. In some cases, this requirement may not align with the patient's actual prognosis and may limit their access to hospice care.

Additionally, the Hospice Medicare benefit requires that the patient give up certain treatments, such as curative care, to receive the benefit. This can be difficult for some patients and their families, who may feel that they are giving up hope in exchange for financial support.

Overall, the Hospice Medicare benefit is a valuable resource for patients and their families facing a terminal illness. It provides financial support for hospice care and access to a team of healthcare professionals who specialize in end-of-life care. However, it is vital for patients and their families to carefully consider the pros and cons of the Hospice Medicare benefit and to make an informed decision about whether it is the right choice for them.

The benefits of hospice care are numerous. Hospice care can provide relief from pain and other symptoms, emotional and spiritual support, and guidance and support during a difficult time for patients and their families. It can also help them make important decisions about end-of-life care, ultimately improving the quality of life for both patients and their loved ones. Without a doubt, hospice care can be a valuable resource for those facing a terminal illness.

Today, hospice care is provided by a team of healthcare professionals, including doctors, nurses, social workers, chaplains, and volunteers. Hospice care can be provided in a variety of settings, including the patient's home, a hospice center, or a nursing home. Hospice care focuses on providing comfort and support, rather than attempting to cure the patient's illness. It is a holistic approach that addresses the physical, emotional, spiritual, and social needs of the patient and their family.

The Hospice Team

One of the primary components of hospice care is the involvement of a multidisciplinary team of healthcare professionals. This team typically includes doctors, nurses, social workers, chaplains, and volunteers, who work together to provide comprehensive care to patients and their families.

One point that must be brought up (seriously, they'll kill me if I don't...), is that no hospice team would be complete without an exceptional administrative staff. The administrative team works mainly behind the scenes in the office, although sometimes even on the road, to ensure that the hospice care team is well-organized and supported. Their efforts are sometimes left unrecognized; however, I can assure you that they are greatly appreciated and their contribution to good patient care does not go unnoticed. The administrative team's attention to detail and ability to juggle multiple tasks at once is essential to the smooth operation of the hospice care team. I owe much of my success to the efforts of the office team (I'm looking at you, Angel... SIR).

> *Pro-Tip: A good case manager will make sure they pop in to say hi to all administrative and leadership team members when they visit the office. A great case manager comes bearing coffee and donuts (or tacos... whatevs).*

Allowing pets in the office can have many benefits for both the employees and the company. Studies have shown that having pets in the workplace can reduce stress, increase morale and productivity, and even lead to better overall mental and physical health for employees.

Having a dog in the office when I visited for supplies or IDG meetings always made my day better. I'll never forget sweet Uma warmly greeting me every time I brought my friend Angel admission paperwork (100% on time every time of course). My day was always instantly improved when I got to spend a little time with Uma.

For many people, their pets are an integral part of their daily lives and bring them a great deal of joy and companionship. Being able to bring their pets to work can help reduce the sense of separation and longing that many people feel when they are away from their furry friends for long periods of time.

In my experience, working with my dog Buttercup has been an absolute joy. Not only does she bring me happiness and comfort throughout the day, but she also helps to create a friendly and welcoming atmosphere in the office. The presence of a pet can help to break the ice and facilitate social interactions among coworkers, leading to stronger team bonds and better overall collaboration.

In short, allowing pets in the office can have numerous benefits for both the employees and the company. Whether it's the stress-reducing effects of petting a furry friend or the sense of community that their presence can create, there's no denying the positive impact that pets can have in the workplace.

The use of pets in hospice care can be a valuable addition to the care plan, helping to provide comfort and support for patients and their families during a difficult time.

I had the great fortune to see Jake the dog in action. Jake was a beloved therapy dog who provided comfort and support to hospice patients and their families. Jake was known for his calm and gentle demeanor, and his ability to sense when someone needed a comforting presence.

Jake worked with a hospice case manager, visiting patients in their homes and in hospice facilities. He would often lay quietly by a patient's side, providing comfort and a sense of companionship. Jake was also known to bring joy and laughter to patients and their families and was often able to lift their spirits during difficult times.

In addition to his work with hospice patients, Jake was involved in community outreach and education. He would visit schools and nursing homes and participate in fundraising events for the hospice organization.

Jake's work as a hospice dog had a profound impact on the lives of those he served. He provided comfort, companionship, and joy to patients and their families, and helped to make their end-of-life experiences more bearable. Jake's legacy lives on through the many lives he touched, and the memories he left behind.

That said, the following professionals are found on most hospice care teams:

Volunteer Coordinator

Volunteer coordinators play a vital role in coordinating community resources for patients and their families. They work to connect patients with volunteers and community resources that can provide support and assistance during a difficult time.

One of the main responsibilities of a volunteer coordinator is to identify and recruit volunteers who are willing and able to provide various types of support to patients and their families. This may include volunteers who are trained in hospice care and can provide companionship, transportation, or other types of assistance to patients. The coordinator may also recruit volunteers who can provide specialized services, such as pet therapy or music therapy, to help improve the patient's quality of life.

In addition to recruiting volunteers, the coordinator is also responsible for coordinating and scheduling volunteer shifts and ensuring that there is sufficient coverage to meet the needs of patients and their families. They may also provide training and support to volunteers to ensure that they are prepared and able to provide the highest level of care to patients.

The volunteer coordinator also plays an important role in coordinating with community resources to ensure that patients and their families have access to the support and assistance they need. This may include connecting patients with local organizations or resources that can provide financial assistance, legal services, or other types of support.

Community Liaison

The role of a hospice *Community Liaison* is to serve as a liaison between the hospice team and the patient's community and to help facilitate communication and coordination between these two groups. The Liaison is often the first to meet a patient and their family and will usually obtain signatures on essential documents needed to admit the patient to hospice services. They will explain the hospice benefit to the patient and family and help them to understand their decision and choices.

Throughout a patient's time on hospice services, the Liaison may also continue to aid communication between the interdisciplinary team members, the patient, and their family depending on their needs. They will also build and maintain relationships with healthcare facilities, hospitals, and other healthcare professionals and organizations.

The Liaison is often the first person a Case Manager can rely on to get a provider's direct phone number or to help get a document signed. They know when the doctors are on vacation, when their kids' birthdays are, where they hide in facilities, and how to get a hold of them quickly.

In addition to serving as a liaison between the hospice team and the patient's community, a Hospice Community Liaison may also coordinate the delivery of hospice services. This may involve coordinating with other hospice team members to ensure that patients receive the care and support they need and working with the patient and their family to develop a care plan tailored to their individual needs.

The liaison is often the first member of the healthcare team to build a relationship with the patient and their family. As a result, they are a trusted and essential member of the team, and the patient and family often rely on them for support and guidance. It is important for the case manager and the liaison to communicate regularly to ensure that the patient's needs are being met efficiently.

The goal of marketing for the Liaison is to increase awareness of hospice care and the services that are available and to help ensure that patients and their families have access to the care and support they need. By promoting the hospice and its services to the patient's community, a Hospice Community Liaison can help to increase the number of patients who are able to access hospice care and can help to ensure that patients and their families are aware of the support and resources that are available to them.

In addition to providing information, a hospice community liaison may also work to change negative misperceptions about hospice care by dispelling common myths and misconceptions. For example, some people may believe that hospice is only for people who are near death, or that it is "giving up" on treatment. A hospice community liaison can help to clarify that hospice is a type of palliative care that is focused on providing comfort and support to individuals and their families during the end of life, and that it can be provided alongside curative treatment.

To effectively market the hospice and its services, a Hospice Community Liaison may need to develop a marketing plan that outlines the specific strategies and tactics that will be used to promote the hospice and its services to the patient's community. This may include developing marketing materials, such as brochures, flyers, and posters, and implementing outreach and informational campaigns to educate the community about hospice care and the services that are available.

As a Case Manager, you may have the chance to attend various events and activities. This can be a great way to get to know the staff at the facility and important community members. These events can also provide valuable networking opportunities for nurses looking to advance their careers. Plus, many marketing professionals want to impress their audience, so they often provide delicious food and refreshments at these events.

> *Pro-Tip: It is widely accepted among ethics committees that accepting gifts in exchange for business favors is unethical. However, there is a loophole that allows the acceptance of perishable items, such as food. Volunteering to help the liaison or marketers in the healthcare field can provide an opportunity to network and gather useful business contacts, as well as getting a full stomach. For a career nurse, forming a relationship with a liaison or marketer can be a valuable asset, especially for those who frequently forget to bring their own lunch.*

Chaplain

Hospice *Chaplains* are healthcare professionals who are trained to provide spiritual and emotional support to patients and their families during a time of terminal illness. They work to meet the spiritual and emotional needs of patients and families, regardless of their religious beliefs or spiritual traditions practices and may work with patients and their loved ones to explore a wide range of spiritual and religious traditions. The role of a Hospice Chaplain is to help patients and their loved one's cope with the emotional and spiritual challenges that often arise during the end-of-life process.

One of the primary roles of chaplains in hospice is to provide spiritual counsel and guidance to patients and their loved ones. This may involve leading prayer or meditation sessions, providing religious sacraments, or simply offering a listening ear and a supportive presence. Chaplains may also work with patients and families to help them find meaning and purpose in their lives as they near the end of life.

> *One of the great chaplains I have been fortunate to work with, and my friend, Gilbert Salgado M.Div., M.A.C.M., has this to say, "The most important thing a chaplain can do regardless of if the patient has a faith or not, is to always be present."*

In addition to providing spiritual support, chaplains in hospice also work closely with other members of the hospice care team to coordinate care for patients. This may involve communicating with doctors, nurses, and other healthcare professionals about the patient's spiritual needs and preferences and working with them to ensure that these needs are being met. Chaplains may also work with social workers and other members of the hospice team to provide support to patients and their families during this challenging time.

A hospice case manager can support and coordinate care with the chaplain in several ways. First, they can facilitate communication between the chaplain and the patient, ensuring that the patient's spiritual and emotional needs are being met. This may involve setting up meetings between the chaplain and the patient, or simply making sure that the chaplain is aware of the patient's spiritual beliefs and preferences.

The hospice case manager can also work with the chaplain to develop a care plan that considers the patient's spiritual needs. This might include identifying any specific rituals or practices that the patient wishes to participate in or coordinating with the chaplain to provide spiritual support to the patient and their family.

In addition, the hospice case manager can help to ensure that the chaplain has access to the necessary resources and support to provide spiritual care to the patient. This may include coordinating with other members of the hospice team, such as nurses and social workers, to provide a supportive environment for the patient's spiritual needs.

When chaplains are unfamiliar with a patient's religious needs, or unable to perform certain ceremonies, they may refer to spiritual leaders in the community. This is most often the case with Catholic and Jewish patients. The case manager can help support the chaplain by networking with other healthcare professionals and maintaining a list of community resources they encounter in their day.

For example, a case manager can introduce themselves to a Catholic Priest who is performing last rites in a facility or hospital. Most Priests will have a business card that you can exchange for yours. This serves the dual purpose of giving the priest's church the name of a hospice company that employs a professional nurse such as yourself. I promise, both your Chaplain and your Community Liaison will greatly appreciate your efforts.

> *Pro-Tip: A good hospice nurse will never forget that they are on stage every time they are in public. They represent not only themselves and the hospice provider they work for but the nursing and hospice fields themselves. Be you but be the best version of yourself.*

Emotional support is a crucial aspect of end-of-life care, and a hospice chaplain is trained to provide this support to the dying patient and their family. The chaplain's role is to listen, offer comfort, and provide a safe and supportive environment for the patient and their loved ones to share their thoughts, feelings, and concerns.

> *"That is the most powerful thing a chaplain can do for a patient and family,"* says Gilbert, *"is to be present with them no matter what the situation is."*

The chaplain may engage in one-on-one conversations with the patient and their family, or lead group discussions to provide a forum for individuals to express their emotions and seek support from others. They may also use therapeutic techniques, such as reflective listening, to help the patient and their loved ones process their feelings and find meaning and purpose during this difficult time.

Bereavement Counselor

A hospice *Bereavement Counselor* provides support and counseling to patients, their families, and other loved ones after the death of a patient. The role of a Hospice Bereavement Counselor is to help individuals cope with the grief and loss associated with the death of a loved one and to provide support and guidance as they navigate the grieving process. It is often a member of the chaplain team or a social worker who performs this role or may involve more members of the team if there is complicated grieving or other challenging aspects of the death.

One of the primary responsibilities of a Hospice Bereavement Counselor is to provide individual and group counseling to patients, their families, and other loved ones who are grieving the loss of a patient. This may involve offering support and guidance as individuals process their emotions and cope with the challenges of dealing with grief and loss and providing resources and support to help them navigate the grieving process. Bereavement Counselors may also provide services and support to facility staff as needed.

In addition to providing individual and group counseling, a Hospice Bereavement Counselor may also be responsible for coordinating bereavement support services within the hospice team. This may involve working with other members of the hospice team to develop and implement bereavement support programs and coordinating with community organizations and other resources to ensure that patients, their families, and other loved ones have access to the support and resources they need.

Hospice bereavement counselors may use a variety of therapeutic approaches to help individuals cope with grief and loss. These may include techniques such as grief education, grief groups, and expressive therapy, which can provide a safe and supportive environment for individuals to process their emotions and find meaning and purpose in their loss.

It is also important for hospice bereavement counselors to be culturally sensitive and aware of the diverse needs of patients and their families. Grief and bereavement can be experienced differently by different cultures and communities, and bereavement counselors need to be attuned to these differences and provide support that is responsive to the specific needs and cultural backgrounds of their clients.

Social Worker

The role of a hospice *Social Worker* is to help patients and their families cope with the social and emotional challenges that often arise during the end-of-life process. The Hospice Social Worker often works closely with the Case Manager to coordinate the delivery of care and support to patients and their families.

One of the primary responsibilities of a Hospice Social Worker is to provide emotional support and counseling to patients and their families. This may involve listening and providing empathy and compassion to patients and their loved ones and helping them to process their emotions and cope with the challenges of dealing with a terminal illness. Hospice Social Workers are trained to provide emotional support in a non-judgmental and compassionate manner and will work with patients and their families to help them navigate the complex emotions that often arise during the end-of-life process.

Helping patients and their loved ones to navigate the practical and logistical aspects of end-of-life care can be an important part of the hospice social worker's role. This may involve coordinating with healthcare providers to ensure that patients receive the medical care and support they need and working with patients and their loved ones to develop a care plan that meets their individual needs and preferences.

In addition to coordinating with healthcare providers, hospice social workers may also assist patients and their families with making funeral arrangements and managing financial and legal affairs. This may include helping individuals to select a funeral home and plan the details of the funeral or memorial service, and assisting with the preparation of legal documents, such as wills and power of attorney documents.

Managing financial and legal affairs can be especially challenging for patients and their families during the end-of-life journey, as they may be dealing with significant emotional and logistical stresses. Hospice social workers can provide valuable support and guidance in this area by helping individuals to understand their options and make informed decisions about their care and financial affairs.

Helping patients and their loved ones to navigate the practical and logistical aspects of end-of-life care can be an important part of the hospice social worker's role. This may involve coordinating with healthcare providers to ensure that patients receive the medical care and support they need and working with patients and their loved ones to develop a care plan that meets their individual needs and preferences.

Home Health Aide

A hospice *Home Health Aide* is a healthcare professional who works as part of a hospice team to provide hands-on care and support to terminally ill patients who are receiving hospice care at home. The role of a Hospice Home Health Aide is to assist patients with activities of daily living, such as bathing, dressing, and grooming, and to provide support and assistance with other tasks as needed, to ensure that their physical and emotional needs are met.

In addition to providing hands-on care and support, a Hospice Home Health Aide may also be responsible for monitoring the patient's condition and providing updates to the Hospice Case Manager. This may involve observing the patient's symptoms and vital signs and reporting any changes or concerns to the Hospice Case Manager. The Hospice Case Manager, in turn, is responsible for coordinating the delivery of care and support to the patient and may work with the Hospice Home Health Aide to ensure that the patient is receiving the care and support they need.

Aides typically see patients on a regular basis and may visit the patient's home daily, weekly, or as needed. The frequency of visits will depend on the patient's individual needs and the care plan that has been developed by the hospice team. Home Health Aides do not typically administer medication, as this is the responsibility of the patient's caregiver or nurse.

Hospice Home Health Aides are a valuable and integral part of the hospice team and are essential to ensuring that patients who are receiving hospice care at home have access to the care and support they need. Home Health Aides work hard to provide compassionate and respectful care to patients and play a crucial role in helping patients and their families cope with the challenges of dealing with a terminal illness. Home Health Aides are dedicated to providing high-quality care to patients and are an invaluable resource to the hospice team.

The case manager plays a crucial role in managing the work of the Hospice Home Health Aide and is responsible for coordinating the delivery of care and support to the patient, and for ensuring that the Home Health Aide has the support and resources they need to provide high-quality care to the patient. Hospice Home Health Aides are hardworking and dedicated professionals who are an essential part of the hospice team, and who play a crucial role in helping patients and their families cope with the challenges of dealing with a terminal illness. They are truly the backbone of good hospice care.

Pro-Tip: Thank your aides. They work very hard.

The Doctor

A doctor's role on a hospice team is to provide medical care and support to patients who are in the end stages of a terminal illness. The doctor works closely with the hospice team, including the Case Manager, to coordinate and manage the patient's care.

Some examples of a doctor's responsibilities on a hospice team may include prescribing medications to manage symptoms and improve the patient's quality of life; making certifying and recertifying visits to patients in their homes and facilities; coordinating care with other members of the hospice team, including the case manager, nurse practitioners, and other healthcare professionals; and communicating with the patient's family and other caregivers to provide support and education.

The doctor and case manager work closely together to coordinate and manage the patient's care. The case manager is responsible for coordinating and managing the overall care of the patient, while the doctor is responsible for providing medical care and treatment in the form of orders for treatment and medication, as well as guidance for the medical care of the patient.

The doctor may see the patient during home visits or at a hospice facility. In some locations, the hospice doctor may delegate certain tasks and visits to a nurse practitioner, who is a healthcare professional with advanced training in nursing.

Sometimes, a *Nurse Practitioner* will be on the hospice team, and they will work closely with the doctor and other members of the hospice team to provide medical care and support to the patient. They may perform recertification visits, physical exams, order and interpret diagnostic tests, prescribe medications, and provide patient education.

A *recertification visit* is a routine visit that occurs every few months to assess the patient's condition and determine their continued eligibility for hospice care. During the visit, the doctor, nurse practitioner, or other appropriate healthcare professional, will assess the patient's condition and determine whether their terminal illness has progressed to the point where they are still eligible for hospice care.

A *Certificate of Terminal Illness* is a document that is completed by a doctor and certifies that the patient has a terminal diagnosis and is expected to have a life expectancy of six months or less if the terminal diagnosis runs its normal course. This document is required for the patient to qualify for hospice care.

A *terminal diagnosis* is a medical term used to describe a condition or disease that cannot be cured and is expected to result in death. It is a serious and often difficult diagnosis for patients and their families to receive, as it signifies the end of life.

The doctor's role in assigning a terminal diagnosis is to provide accurate and thorough information about the patient's condition, prognosis, and treatment options. This may involve reviewing the patient's medical history, performing physical examinations, ordering diagnostic tests, and consulting with other healthcare professionals as needed. It is often the RN Case Manager who collects the past medical history and provides this to the doctor who will then use the information to provide a terminal diagnosis.

> *Pro Tip: Doctors greatly appreciate a thorough, yet concise, past medical history. You should ask the doctor if they have a template that they would prefer you to use when providing this information to them. Doctors frequently have caseloads of dozens or more patients and must review the information quickly, therefore accuracy and completeness will earn you great favor from them.*

When a doctor provides a terminal diagnosis, they are stating that the patient's illness is incurable, and that death is imminent. To make this determination, the doctor will review a number of criteria, including:

- The patient's medical history: This includes any previous diagnoses, treatments, and responses to treatment.

- The patient's current symptoms: The doctor will consider the severity and frequency of the patient's symptoms, as well as how they are affecting the patient's quality of life.

- The results of diagnostic tests: The doctor may order a range of tests to help confirm the diagnosis and determine the extent of the illness. These might include imaging tests, such as CT scans or MRIs, or laboratory tests, such as blood tests or biopsies.

- The patient's prognosis: The doctor will consider the likelihood of the patient's condition improving or worsening over time, as well as the potential for complications.

- The patient's preferences: The doctor will also take into account the patient's wishes and values, including their feelings about further treatment and their end-of-life goals.

It should be noted that a terminal diagnosis is not a death sentence. While it means that the patient's condition is incurable, it does not mean that they will not receive treatment to manage their symptoms and improve their quality of life. Additionally, the prognosis for a terminal illness can change over time, so the doctor will continue to monitor the patient and adjust the treatment plan as needed.

Some common terminal diagnoses that may be seen in hospice care include advanced cancer, end-stage heart disease, advanced dementia, and advanced lung disease. Other terminal conditions may include kidney failure, liver failure, advanced HIV/AIDS, and failure-to-thrive.

A note on pursuing Failure-to-Thrive as a terminal diagnosis: Failure-to-thrive (FTT) is a term used to describe a condition in which a person, particularly an infant or elderly individual, experiences a significant decline in physical and/or cognitive function. FTT can be caused by a variety of factors, including underlying medical conditions, malnutrition, and social or environmental issues.

In some cases, failure-to-thrive may be used as a terminal diagnosis in hospice care, particularly for elderly individuals who have experienced a significant decline in function and are no longer responding to treatment. In these cases, the goal of hospice care may be to manage the patient's symptoms and improve their quality of life, rather than to attempt to reverse the underlying condition.

However, failure-to-thrive is not always a terminal diagnosis and treatment may be successful in some cases. For example, a patient with FTT due to malnutrition may be able to recover with proper nutrition and medical care. Therefore, healthcare providers must carefully assess each patient's specific circumstances and past medical history to determine the most appropriate course of treatment. For this reason, a medical doctor will only assign a terminal diagnosis following a thorough review of the patient's medical history and after the patient has provided informed consent about their decision to accept end-of-life care versus curative or life-extending treatment.

Two other tools utilized by the doctor and hospice care team for evaluating a patient's condition include the FAST scale and the PPS scale.

The *FAST (Functional Assessment Staging)* scale is a tool used to evaluate the functional status and cognitive abilities of a patient with dementia. It is commonly used in hospice care to determine the appropriate level of care and to set goals for care. The FAST scale has five stages, ranging from no impairment to severe impairment. Each stage is based on the patient's ability to perform activities of daily living, such as bathing, dressing, and using the toilet.

1. No cognitive or functional difficulties are present.

2. The person may complain of forgetting the location of objects or have difficulty finding words, but these issues do not affect their daily functioning.

3. There is a noticeable decline in job performance and the person may have difficulty navigating to new locations or organizing tasks.

4. The person has trouble completing complex tasks such as planning a dinner party or managing their personal finances.

5. The person requires assistance in selecting appropriate clothing for the day, season, or occasion, and may wear the same clothing repeatedly without supervision.

6. A: The person occasionally or more frequently has difficulty properly dressing themselves, such as putting street clothes on over pajamas, wearing shoes on the wrong feet, or struggling to button clothing.

   B: The person may have trouble bathing properly, such as adjusting the water temperature or difficulty with personal hygiene.

   C: The person may have issues with toileting, such as forgetting to flush the toilet, improper wiping, or difficulty disposing of toilet tissue.

   D. The person may experience urinary incontinence occasionally or more frequently.

   E: The person may experience fecal incontinence occasionally or more frequently.

7. A: The person can only speak a few different intelligible words in an average day or during an intensive interview.

   B: The person can only speak a single intelligible word in an average day or during an intensive interview.

   C: The person is unable to walk without assistance.

   D: The person cannot sit up without assistance.

   E: The person is unable to smile.

   F: The person is unable to hold their head up independently.

The *Palliative Performance Scale (PPS)* is a tool used to assess the functional status and overall performance of a patient with a terminal illness. It is used to evaluate the patient's physical and cognitive abilities, including their ability to walk, dress, bathe, and eat, as well as their ability to communicate and interact with others. The PPS scale ranges from 0 to 100, with a score of 0 indicating that the patient is completely bedridden and unable to perform any activities of daily living, and a score of 100 indicating that the patient is fully functional and able to perform all activities of daily living without any assistance. The PPS scale is typically used by hospice care teams to assess the patient's prognosis and determine the appropriate level of care. It is also used to monitor the patient's progress and adjust the care plan as needed.

100%   - Full ambulation
       - Normal activity and work / No evidence of disease
       - Full self-care
       - Normal intake
       - Full consciousness

90%   - Full ambulation
       - Normal activity and work / Some evidence of disease
       - Full self-care
       - Normal intake
       - Full consciousness

80%   - Full ambulation
       - Normal activity and work / Some evidence of disease
       - Full self-care
       - Normal or reduced intake
       - Full consciousness

Patients below this level are generally considered appropriate for a hospice evaluation:

70%   - Reduced ambulation
       - Unable to do normal job or work / Significant disease
       - Full self-care
       - Normal or reduced intake
       - Full consciousness

60%   - Reduced ambulation
       - Unable to do hobby or housework / Significant disease
       - Occasional assistance necessary
       - Normal or reduced intake
       - Full consciousness / confusion

50%	- Mainly sit/lie
	- Unable to do any work / Extensive disease
	- Considerable assistance required
	- Normal or reduced intake
	- Full consciousness / confusion

50% - Mainly sit/lie
     - Unable to do any work / Extensive disease
     - Considerable assistance required
     - Normal or reduced intake
     - Full consciousness / confusion

40% - Mainly in bed
     - Unable to do most activity / Extensive disease
     - Mainly assistance
     - Normal or reduced intake
     - Full or drowsy consciousness +/- confusion

30% - Totally bedbound
     - Unable to do any activity / Extensive disease
     - Total care
     - Normal or reduced intake
     - Full or drowsy consciousness +/- confusion

20% - Totally bedbound
     - Unable to do any activity / Extensive disease
     - Total care
     - Minimal to sips
     - Full or drowsy consciousness +/- confusion

10% - Totally bedbound
     - Unable to do any activity / Extensive disease
     - Total care
     - Mouth care only
     - Full or drowsy consciousness +/- confusion

0%   - Death

RNCM: The Nurse Case Manager

At the heart of the hospice care team is the Case Manager *brushes off shoulder*. The hospice case manager is responsible for coordinating and overseeing the care of hospice patients and ensuring that their needs are met in a timely and effective manner. This includes developing and implementing a care plan, coordinating with other members of the hospice care team, and communicating with patients and their families.

To be a successful hospice case manager, a nurse must have a variety of skills and qualities. These include strong communication and interpersonal skills, the ability to work well in a team, and the ability to handle complex and emotional situations. They must also have a thorough understanding of the principles of hospice care and be able to apply this knowledge in a practical and compassionate manner.

Communication is a central part of the hospice case manager's role. They must be able to effectively communicate with patients and their families, providing them with information about their care, answering their questions, and addressing their concerns. They must also be able to communicate effectively with other members of the hospice care team, sharing information and coordinating care.

One of the main responsibilities of the hospice case manager is to develop and implement a comprehensive care plan for each patient. The care plan is the foundation of the case manager's work. It is a roadmap for their patient's care and should be developed with input from the patient, their family, and the rest of the hospice care team. This care plan should be tailored to the individual needs of the patient and should be regularly reviewed and updated to ensure that it continues to meet their changing needs.

The care plan should include goals and objectives for the patient's care, as well as a detailed plan for achieving those goals. It should also include a plan for managing symptoms and pain, as well as a plan for providing emotional and spiritual support to the patient and their family.

The case manager is responsible for coordinating with other members of the hospice care team to ensure that the plan is implemented effectively. The hospice case manager is responsible for ensuring that all team members are aware of the patient's care plan and are working towards the same goals. This may involve communicating with team members about the patient's progress, coordinating the delivery of medical care, and facilitating communication between team members.

Pro-Tip: A hospice case manager cannot successfully provide good care without their team. Be a team player. Also, allow your team to do their job. Do not assume the role of the social worker or chaplain in the heat of the moment. A good case manager knows when to put a time-out on a situation and call on a member of their team to assist.

In addition to coordinating care, the hospice case manager should also be available to answer questions and provide support to team members as needed. They should be able to identify any potential challenges or issues that may arise in the patient's care and work with the team to develop solutions.

In addition to care planning and coordination, the hospice case manager is also responsible for conducting clinical assessments of patients, identifying and managing symptoms and pain, and providing emotional and spiritual support.

To conduct a thorough clinical assessment, the hospice case manager should complete a physical examination of the patient, assess their symptoms and pain levels, and review their medical history. They should also assess the patient's emotional and spiritual well-being and provide support as needed.

Managing symptoms and pain is a key part of the hospice case manager's role. This may involve administering medications, providing comfort measures, or making referrals to other members of the hospice care team. Managing symptoms and pain can be challenging, but it is a crucial part of hospice care.

In addition to providing physical support, the hospice case manager should also provide emotional and spiritual support to patients and their families. This may involve listening to their concerns, providing comfort and reassurance, and helping them to find meaning and purpose in their remaining time together.

The role of the hospice case manager is complex and challenging, but also incredibly rewarding. By providing comprehensive care planning, coordination, and clinical support, the hospice case manager plays a vital role in ensuring that patients and their families receive the high-quality care they deserve.

To help facilitate the coordination of care and communication, hospice providers will hold regular *interdisciplinary team (IDT)* or *interdisciplinary group (IDG) meetings*. The IDT/IDG is a meeting of the hospice team that is held to discuss the care and management of patients who are receiving hospice services.

The IDT/IDG typically includes all hospice care team members who meet at regular intervals to collaborate on how to provide comprehensive care to their patients and families. During the IDT/IDG meeting, team members discuss the progress of each patient, review their care plans, and identify any issues or concerns that need to be addressed. The IDT/IDG may also review new patient referrals and develop care plans for newly admitted patients.

IDT/IDG meetings are typically held weekly or monthly and may last for several hours. These meetings provide an opportunity for team members to share information and ideas, and to learn from each other's experiences and expertise. IDT/IDG meetings can be a valuable source of support and education for nurses and other healthcare professionals. They provide an opportunity to learn from colleagues and to stay up to date on best practices and emerging trends in hospice care.

IDT/IDG meetings can also be a much-needed source of morale and comradery for team members. They provide an opportunity for team members to connect with each other and share their challenges and triumphs.

> *Pro Tip: Do not underestimate the lonely feelings that creep up in even the most introverted nurse when spending most of your time practicing autonomously. It is important for nurses to collaborate with other healthcare professionals regularly to avoid feelings of isolation, imposter syndrome, or other negative effects that come along with remote work. Even group phone or video calls can help. Make friends on your team that you can rely on when you need to vent or just talk.*

IDT/IDG meetings are also a good opportunity for team members to pick up supplies for patient visits, including wound care supplies and other necessary items. *Car-stock* is a term used to describe a supply of medications and other supplies that are kept in a vehicle for use during patient visits. Car-stock supplies are typically replenished at IDT/IDG meetings or other scheduled times.

In conclusion, hospice care is a specialized form of healthcare that focuses on providing comfort and support to individuals with terminal illnesses and their loved ones during the end-of-life journey. With a history dating back to ancient time, hospice care has evolved into a widely respected and integral part of the healthcare system, providing comprehensive and compassionate care to millions of individuals and their families each year.

One of the main benefits of hospice care is that it focuses on the overall well-being of the patient, rather than just their physical symptoms. Hospice care teams provide a range of services, including medical care, emotional support, and spiritual guidance, to help individuals find meaning and purpose during this difficult time. Additionally, hospice care can be provided in a variety of settings, including patients' homes, hospitals, and hospice facilities, allowing individuals to receive care in the location of their choice.

Overall, hospice care is an important resource for individuals with terminal illnesses and their loved ones, providing compassionate and comprehensive care during the end-of-life journey.

Chapter 2

The Role of the Hospice Case Manager

I was sitting on my couch, feeling burnt out and overwhelmed by my job as a private-duty pediatric nurse. Most of my week was spent working in a hostile high-school environment that frequently triggered my PTSD, and I was feeling depressed and discouraged. As I sat there, staring at the wall, trying to come up with a plan, I received a message from my former nursing school classmate Carrie.

She knew that I was struggling to find a nursing role that I felt good about, and she suggested that I apply for a position as an RN Case Manager at the hospice provider she had done her clinical rotations during school. At first, I was hesitant. I wasn't sure if I was ready to make such a big change, and I wasn't sure if I had the right skills or experience to work in hospice care. But as I thought about it, I remembered that I was a nurse and my skills would translate, so I decided to take a chance and apply for the job.

After a brief interview period, I was offered the position which I eagerly accepted. I was excited to start this new chapter in my career, and I was eager to see what hospice care had to offer.

As I began my new job, I was immediately struck by the rewarding nature of providing end-of-life care. I found that working with patients and their families at such a difficult time was incredibly fulfilling, and I was touched by the deep sense of gratitude and appreciation that I received from my clients.

I quickly realized that hospice care was exactly where I belonged, and I was grateful to Carrie for suggesting that I apply for the job. I was able to leave behind the stress and negativity of my previous job, and instead, focus on providing compassionate and comprehensive care to my patients and their loved ones. It was an experience that changed my life, and I will always be grateful for the opportunity to work in hospice care.

Networking with other healthcare professionals has played a crucial role in my career journey. I am grateful to my friend and colleague Carrie who introduced me to the hospice field. She later proved to be one of the best nurses I would ever encounter when I was the Executive Director for an 81-bed memory care community, and I hired her to ~~save my life~~ be my Director of Nursing.

Time and again, colleagues and peers have provided me with more opportunities than I could ever possibly take advantage of. Without these valuable connections, I would not be where I am today, and I wouldn't have the fulfilling healthcare experiences that I am so grateful for. Thank you, Carrie Cadenhead, BSN, RN. Thank you, Simeon Purkey, MA. Thank you, Wendy Chaston, RN. Thank you, Katie Brown, RN for being my first hospice preceptor. And thank you to so many others for your invaluable contributions to my professional journey.

Pro-Tip: Always thank your spouse too. Thanks, wife!

As a primary member of the hospice care team, the hospice case manager plays a crucial role in ensuring that patients with terminal illnesses receive the highest quality of care possible. They are responsible for coordinating and overseeing all aspects of a patient's care, including managing the care provided by other members of the hospice team, coordinating communication between the patient and their healthcare providers, and ensuring that the patient's physical, emotional, and spiritual needs are met.

In addition to managing the patient's care, the hospice case manager also serves as an advocate for the patient and their family, working to ensure that their rights and wishes are respected and that they receive the support they need during this difficult time. The hospice case manager is a vital member of the hospice care team, and their expertise and dedication are essential in helping patients and their families navigate the challenges of a terminal illness.

> *"The hospice case manager is the heart of the hospice care team," says Olga Kutselyk, RN, a hospice nurse with over 10 years of nursing experience. "They are the ones who ensure that everything runs smoothly and that our patients receive the best possible care."*

The specific responsibilities of the hospice case manager may vary depending on the setting and the individual needs of the patient. However, some common responsibilities include:

- Developing and implementing a comprehensive care plan for each patient

- Coordinating with other members of the hospice care team, including doctors, nurses, social workers, and volunteers

- Communicating with patients and their families, providing them with information about their care, and answering their questions

- Conducting clinical assessments of patients, including physical examinations, symptom and pain management assessments, and emotional and spiritual assessments

- Providing symptom and pain management, including administering medications and providing comfort measures

- Providing emotional and spiritual support to patients and their families

"The hospice case manager has a lot of responsibilities, but they are all important in providing high-quality care to our patients," says Kutselyk. "Without the hospice case manager, the hospice care team would not be able to function effectively."

To be a successful hospice case manager, a nurse must have a variety of skills and qualities. These include strong communication and interpersonal skills, the ability to work well in a team, and the ability to handle complex and emotional situations. They must also have a thorough understanding of the principles of hospice care and be able to apply this knowledge in a practical and compassionate manner.

"Working as a hospice case manager requires a special set of skills and qualities," says Kutselyk. "It is not a job for everyone, but for those who are well-suited to it, it can be incredibly rewarding."

Some specific skills and qualities that are essential for the hospice case manager include:

Strong communication skills

Effective *communication skills* are critical for hospice nurses to be able to provide top-quality care to their patients. As a hospice nurse, you will be responsible for communicating with patients and their families, keeping them informed about their care, answering their questions, and addressing their concerns. In addition, you will need to communicate with other members of the hospice care team, such as doctors, social workers, and volunteers, to coordinate and manage the care of your patients.

Strong communication skills are essential for hospice nurses to be able to effectively connect with their patients and families, understand their needs, and provide the support and comfort they need during this challenging time. In addition to these verbal communication skills, hospice nurses should also be proficient in nonverbal communication, such as the use of body language and facial expressions, to effectively connect with their patients and convey empathy and compassion.

Effective communication involves not only speaking clearly and accurately to patients and their loved ones but also actively listening to their concerns and needs. This means paying attention to what they are saying, asking clarifying questions, and showing empathy and understanding of their situation.

The hospice nurse should approach the patient with a compassionate and caring tone, showing empathy, and understanding for the patient's situation. It is important for the nurse to be open and honest with the patient and to discuss the patient's prognosis in a straightforward and clear manner, while also being sensitive to the patient's feelings and needs.

It can be difficult to know how to respond to questions about a patient's prognosis, as it can be a sensitive and emotional topic for both the patient and their family. A common response, albeit emotionless and somewhat insensitive, is to say, "There is no crystal ball." It is important for the hospice nurse to be honest and straightforward with the patient and their family, while also being compassionate and understanding of their feelings. The nurse should approach the conversation with a caring and supportive tone and allow the patient and their family to express their thoughts and feelings.

It is generally best to be honest with the patient and their family about the patient's prognosis, while also emphasizing that they are receiving the best possible care and support. The nurse can also reassure the patient and their family that they will be there to help them through this difficult time. It may also be helpful for the nurse to offer resources such as counseling or support groups to help the patient and their family cope with the situation.

The most important thing to tell a dying patient will vary depending on the individual and their specific circumstances. However, there are some general points that the hospice nurse may want to communicate to the patient:

- You are not alone: It is important for the patient to know that they are being cared for and that they are not alone in this difficult time.

- Your feelings and wishes matter: The nurse should respect the patient's feelings and wishes and do their best to address any concerns or requests that the patient may have.

- You will be kept comfortable: The nurse should reassure the patient that their comfort is a priority and that they will do everything possible to manage any pain or other symptoms that the patient may be experiencing.

- **You can still have a sense of control:** Even though the patient may not be able to control the overall outcome of their illness, they can still have a sense of control over other aspects of their care, such as their treatment plan and the people they want to be with. The nurse should encourage the patient to make decisions and express their preferences to the extent that they are able.

- **You are loved:** It is important for the patient to know that they are loved and that their relationships and connections with others are valued. The nurse should encourage the patient to spend time with loved ones and to express their feelings and concerns to them.

The nurse should also consider the patient's cultural and personal beliefs and values, as well as any communication barriers that may exist. It may be helpful for the nurse to ask the patient how they would like to be informed about their prognosis and to involve the patient's family or loved ones in these discussions as appropriate.

To establish trust and rapport with patients and their families, it is important for the case manager to be open and transparent in their communication, sharing information clearly and honestly and addressing any concerns that may arise. It is also important to be responsive to the patient's needs and preferences, tailoring your communication style and approach to suit their individual needs. This can help to create a positive and collaborative relationship, which is essential for providing the best possible care.

You should always ask patients and their families about their communication preferences to ensure that everyone is on the same page and that their needs are being met. This can include asking about their preferred methods of communication, such as phone calls or text messages, as well as how much notification they would like before visits. By taking the time to understand their preferences, you can help to ensure that you are able to effectively communicate with them and provide the best possible care.

The hospice case manager must take an active role in facilitating communication. In the case of patients in long-term care facilities or memory care communities, it is especially important to act as an advocate for your patients and facilitate communication between the patient and the facility as well as their family. This can involve making sure that the facility is aware of the patient's needs and preferences and working to ensure that any issues or concerns are addressed in a timely and effective manner.

Effective communication can help to alleviate the patient's and their family's stress and anxiety and can improve their satisfaction with the care they receive. It can also facilitate the patient's ability to make informed decisions about their care and to communicate their wishes to their healthcare team.

Interpersonal skills

Hospice nurses must also possess excellent *interpersonal skills* to provide the highest quality of care to their patients. This involves being able to build strong, trusting relationships with patients and their families, and providing them with emotional and spiritual support. It also means being able to work well with other members of the hospice care team, collaborating and coordinating care to ensure that the patient's needs are met in a timely and effective manner.

Hospice nurses work with patients and their families during extraordinarily challenging and emotional times in their lives. You will need to be able to establish a strong connection with your patients and build trust and understanding with them. This may involve listening to their concerns and fears, providing them with emotional support and comfort, and helping them to understand their care and treatment options. You should also be able to recognize and respect the cultural and spiritual beliefs of your patients and their families, and to adapt your approach to meet their specific needs and preferences.

Respecting cultural and spiritual beliefs is an important part of providing compassionate and high-quality healthcare. As a hospice nurse, you will likely be working with patients and families from a wide range of cultural and spiritual backgrounds. It is important to be open-minded and respectful of these differences and to be willing to learn about and adapt to the specific needs and preferences of your patients and their families.

This may involve finding ways to incorporate cultural or spiritual practices into their care, such as providing accommodations for prayer or other rituals, or simply being mindful of cultural taboos or sensitivities. By showing respect for your patients' beliefs and traditions, you can help to build trust and establish a strong connection with them, which is essential for providing the best possible care during this challenging and emotional time.

You will also need to be able to work effectively with other members of the hospice care team, including doctors, social workers, and volunteers. This may involve collaborating with these team members to coordinate and oversee the care of your patients and sharing information and resources to ensure that the patient's needs are met in the most effective way possible. Strong interpersonal skills are essential for hospice nurses to be able to build strong working relationships with their colleagues and to provide the best possible care to their patients.

Emotional Intelligence

As a hospice nurse, you will be working with patients who are facing a terminal illness and who may be experiencing a range of emotions, including sadness, fear, anger, and hopelessness. You will need to be able to recognize and understand these emotions, and to provide your patients with the emotional and spiritual support that they need to cope with their illness and their end-of-life journey. This may involve listening to their concerns and fears, providing them with comfort and reassurance, and helping them to understand their care and treatment options.

Emotional intelligence is a critical quality for hospice nurses to possess in order to provide the highest quality of care to their patients. It involves being self-aware, self-regulated, empathetic, and able to effectively communicate and relate to others. In the context of hospice care, this means being able to handle difficult and emotional situations with compassion and professionalism, while also providing support and comfort to patients and their families.

To have high emotional intelligence, hospice nurses must be able to recognize and understand their own emotions, as well as the emotions of their patients and their families. This involves being able to manage their own stress and emotions in a healthy way, as well as being able to sense when patients or families are experiencing strong emotions and responding in a supportive and caring manner.

By developing their emotional intelligence, hospice nurses can better understand and respond to the needs and feelings of their patients and families, ultimately improving the quality of care they are able to provide.

You will also need to be able to maintain a professional and compassionate attitude, even in challenging circumstances. This may involve managing your own emotions and reactions and finding ways to provide support and comfort to your patients and their families without becoming overwhelmed or distressed.

There are several ways that hospice nurses can manage their emotions and reactions when working with patients who are facing a terminal illness:

- Practice self-care: Hospice nurses must prioritize their own well-being and engage in self-care practices to manage the stress and emotions that can come with this work. This may include activities such as getting enough sleep, eating a healthy diet, exercising regularly, and finding ways to relax and destress.

- Seek support: It is normal for hospice nurses to experience a range of emotions when working with patients who are facing a terminal illness. It can be helpful to seek support from colleagues, supervisors, or a mental health professional to process these emotions and to find healthy ways to cope with the challenges of this work.

- Set boundaries: It is imperative for hospice nurses to set healthy boundaries with their patients and their families, and to recognize when they need to take a break or step back from a situation to protect their own well-being.

- Use relaxation techniques: There are a variety of relaxation techniques that hospice nurses can use to manage their emotions and reactions, including deep breathing, meditation, and visualization.

- Seek supervision: Hospice nurses can benefit from regular supervision with a supervisor or mentor to debrief about their work, process their emotions, and receive guidance and support.

By taking care of their own well-being and seeking support when needed, hospice nurses can effectively manage their emotions and reactions, even in the most challenging situations. High emotional intelligence is essential for hospice nurses to be able to provide the care and support that their patients need during this difficult time and to help them navigate the challenges and emotions of terminal illness with grace and dignity.

Knowledge of hospice care

As a hospice case manager, it is important to be the subject-matter-expert in the room when it comes to end-of-life care. This means being a trusted resource and a wealth of knowledge that others can rely on for accurate and timely information. Being well-versed in your craft and having a deep understanding of end-of-life care is essential for being able to provide the best possible care to your patients and their families.

To be an effective hospice case manager, you must be committed to staying up to date on the latest best practices and developments in the field. This may involve continuing your education through professional development courses or staying informed about new research and guidelines. By constantly seeking to improve your knowledge and skills, you can ensure that you are able to provide the most informed and compassionate care to your patients and families. Additionally, by being a reliable source of information and expertise, you can help to ease the burden on patients and their families during this challenging and emotional time and provide them with the support and resources they need to navigate the end-of-life process.

To provide the highest quality of care to their patients, hospice nurses must have a comprehensive understanding of the principles and practices of hospice care and be able to apply this knowledge in a practical and compassionate manner. As a hospice case manager, you will be responsible for providing a range of care services to your patients, including conducting clinical assessments, managing symptoms and pain, and providing emotional and spiritual support.

To be able to effectively provide these services, you will need to have a deep understanding of the principles of hospice care, including symptom and pain management, advanced care planning, and ethical and legal considerations. You will need to be knowledgeable about the various treatment options available to manage symptoms and pain and be able to work with patients and their families to develop care plans that meet their individual needs and preferences.

To provide high-quality care to your patients, it is important to approach your work with compassion, empathy, and a strong sense of professional ethics. This may involve being a supportive presence for your patients and their families, offering emotional and psychological support, and helping them to understand their care and treatment options. You should also be able to recognize and respect the cultural and spiritual beliefs of your patients and their families and adapt your approach to meet their specific needs and preferences. By being compassionate and empathetic, and by providing care that is grounded in the principles and practices of hospice care, you can help to make a difficult and emotional time a little bit easier for your patients and their families.

Flexibility and adaptability

In addition to strong communication, interpersonal, and emotional intelligence skills, hospice case managers must also have strong *flexibility and adaptability*. This means being able to adapt to changing situations and needs and being flexible in your approach to care.

As a hospice nurse, you will be working with patients who are facing a terminal illness, and their needs and circumstances may change rapidly and unexpectedly. You will need to be able to adjust the care plan as needed and to respond to the changing needs and preferences of your patients. This may involve making changes to the treatment plan, coordinating with other members of the care team, and communicating with the patient and their family to ensure that their needs are being met.

You will also need to be able to adapt to different patients and their families and provide care that is tailored to their individual needs and circumstances. This may involve working with patients from different backgrounds, with different cultural and religious beliefs, and with different preferences and priorities. To provide the best possible care to your patients, you will need to be flexible and adaptable, and be able to adjust your approach to meet the unique needs and preferences of each patient.

> "Having the right skills and knowledge are essential for the hospice case manager," says Kutselyk. "Without them, it would be impossible to provide the high-quality care that our patients deserve."

Working as a hospice case manager can be an incredibly fulfilling and rewarding career choice, but it is not without its challenges. Providing hospice care involves a significant emotional and physical investment, and case managers must be prepared to face a range of challenges in their work. These challenges may include dealing with complex medical situations, managing a high workload, and providing emotional support to patients and their families during difficult times. Despite these challenges, many hospice case managers find great meaning and purpose in their work, as they are able to provide compassionate care and support to individuals and families facing terminal illnesses.

Some common challenges faced by hospice case managers, as well as solutions, include:

Managing Symptoms and Pain

Providing *pain control* to a dying patient in hospice care is a crucial aspect of end-of-life care. It is important to alleviate as much suffering as possible and ensure that the patient is comfortable in their final days. There are several ways to approach pain management in hospice care, and the case manager will work closely with the patient and their loved ones, as well as the hospice care team, to determine the most appropriate course of action.

One approach to pain management in hospice care is through the use of medications. Non-opioid pain medications, such as acetaminophen or nonsteroidal anti-inflammatory drugs (NSAIDs), can be effective in relieving mild to moderate pain. Opioids, such as morphine, may be necessary for more severe pain. The hospice nurse must carefully monitor the patient's response to these medications and adjust the dosage as needed.

In addition to medication, other methods of pain management can be used in hospice care. These may include physical therapies such as massage or heat/cold therapy, relaxation techniques such as deep breathing or meditation, and complementary therapies such as music therapy or aromatherapy. Remember to consider the patient's preferences and cultural/spiritual beliefs when selecting pain management techniques.

Some cultures may have specific beliefs about the use of certain medications or may prefer to use natural remedies or spiritual practices to manage pain. The care team must respect these beliefs and work with the patient and their family to find a pain management plan that is consistent with their cultural and spiritual values.

It is also important for the nurse to be open and willing to learn about the patient's cultural and spiritual beliefs, as this can help to build trust and improve the patient's overall experience of care. The nurse should also be aware of any potential language barriers and make sure that there is an appropriate translator available if needed. Many healthcare organizations offer their care team members an 800 number to call for translation services. Additionally, there are many phone apps available that offer free translation services so that the patient can accurately communicate their pain to you and you can offer effective pain management.

The case manager will also address any physical symptoms that may be contributing to the patient's pain, such as constipation or shortness of breath. These symptoms can often be managed through the use of comfort kit medications and other non-pharmacologic therapies.

Comfort kit medications are a set of medications that are commonly used in hospice care to manage symptoms such as pain, nausea, constipation, and anxiety. These medications are usually administered on a regular basis to help keep symptoms under control and to improve the patient's quality of life. Non-pharmacologic therapies, on the other hand, are interventions that do not involve the use of medications. These can include techniques such as massage, relaxation techniques, and guided imagery, which can help to reduce pain and improve overall comfort and well-being.

By addressing physical symptoms and utilizing both pharmacologic and non-pharmacologic therapies as needed, hospice case managers can help to ensure that patients are as comfortable as possible and that their pain is being effectively managed. This is an essential part of providing high-quality end-of-life care.

Effective communication is a crucial aspect of pain management in hospice care. It involves being open and honest with patients about their pain and how it is being managed and involving them in the decision-making process about their care. By engaging in clear and open communication, you can help to ensure that patients are comfortable and that their pain is being managed in a way that meets their needs and preferences.

Effective communication also involves including the patient's loved ones in the care process. This may involve asking them about the patient's pain management preferences or seeking their input on how to provide comfort and support. By involving the patient's loved ones in the care process, you can help to create a sense of teamwork and collaboration, which can be especially important during this challenging and emotional time.

Providing pain control to a dying patient in hospice care requires a proactive, compassionate, and holistic approach that considers the patient's physical, emotional, and spiritual needs. The case manager will work closely with the patient, their loved ones, and the hospice care team to determine the most appropriate pain management plan and to continually assess and adjust the plan as needed.

Providing emotional support

Providing *emotional and spiritual support* to patients and their families is a key aspect of hospice care, and it requires a high level of sensitivity, compassion, and skill. Hospice case managers must be able to handle difficult and emotional situations and provide comfort and support to patients and their families as they navigate the challenges of a terminal illness. They must also be able to provide support to other members of the hospice care team, who may also be dealing with difficult emotions.

One of the challenges of providing emotional support as a hospice case manager is that patients and their families may be experiencing a wide range of emotions, including fear, anxiety, grief, and sadness. These emotions can be difficult to cope with, and hospice case managers must be able to provide support that is appropriate and effective for each individual patient. This may involve listening to patients and families, providing guidance and information, and helping them to cope with their emotions.

Another common challenge that hospice case managers may face is dealing with patients and their families who are resistant to emotional support or hesitant to express their emotions. This can make it difficult for hospice case managers to provide the support that patients and their families need and can lead to misunderstandings or conflicts.

To address this challenge, hospice case managers may need to be proactive in seeking out opportunities to provide support. This may involve being patient and understanding as patients and families navigate their emotions and being willing to listen and provide a supportive presence without judgment or pressure. It may also involve finding creative ways to engage with patients and their families, such as through activities or shared experiences that can help to facilitate emotional expression and connection.

By being proactive and patient, and by being willing to listen and provide support in a non-judgmental way, hospice case managers can help to create a safe and supportive environment for patients and their families, even if they are resistant to emotional support or hesitant to express their emotions. This is an essential part of providing high-quality end-of-life care.

Coordinating care

Coordinating care is a critical aspect of hospice care, and it requires a high level of organizational skills, communication, and collaboration. Hospice case managers must be able to work effectively with other members of the hospice care team, as well as with other healthcare providers, to ensure that patients receive the care they need. They must also be able to manage their own time and workload effectively and prioritize tasks to ensure that patients receive timely and appropriate care.

One of the challenges of coordinating care as a hospice case manager is managing the diverse team of professionals who are responsible for providing hospice care. This team may include doctors, nurses, social workers, and volunteers, each with their own areas of expertise and responsibilities. Coordinating and overseeing the care of patients with such a diverse team can be a complex and challenging task, and it is important for hospice case managers to be able to effectively communicate with all members of the care team and establish clear roles and responsibilities.

To address this challenge, hospice case managers must be skilled at communication and team management. This may involve holding regular meetings with the care team to discuss the patient's progress, coordinating care activities and tasks, and communicating any changes or updates to the patient's plan of care. It may also involve working with the care team to establish clear roles and responsibilities for each member and ensuring that all team members are aware of their responsibilities and are working together effectively.

Another challenge of coordinating hospice care is the fact that patients and their families may have different preferences and priorities, and multiple parties may be involved in the decision-making process. This can make it difficult for hospice case managers to coordinate care and can lead to conflicts or misunderstandings if the needs and preferences of all parties are not taken into account or in agreement.

To address this challenge, hospice case managers must be able to listen to the needs and preferences of patients and families and work with them to develop a care plan that meets their needs and goals. This may involve having open and honest communication with patients and their families, asking questions to better understand their needs and preferences, and being willing to work with them to develop a care plan that meets their specific needs and goals. It may also involve being flexible and willing to make adjustments to the care plan as needed, in order to ensure that it continues to meet the needs and goals of the patient and their family as the patient's condition changes.

By being open and responsive to the needs and preferences of patients and their families, hospice case managers can help to ensure that care is coordinated and that all parties are on the same page, ultimately improving the quality of care and the patient's experience.

Hospice care can be provided in a variety of settings, including the patient's home, a hospice facility, or a hospital. This diversity in care settings can present a challenge for hospice case managers, as it can be difficult to coordinate care and ensure that patients receive consistent and high-quality care.

To address this challenge, hospice case managers must be able to work closely with other members of the care team and establish clear processes and protocols to ensure that care is coordinated and seamless, regardless of the setting. This may involve developing care plans that are specific to the patient's needs and goals, and that take into account the unique features and resources of the care setting. It may also involve working with other members of the care team to ensure that care is coordinated and that all team members are aware of their roles and responsibilities.

By establishing clear processes and protocols and working closely with other members of the care team, hospice case managers can help to ensure that patients receive the highest quality of care, regardless of the setting in which they receive it. This is an important part of providing compassionate and effective end-of-life care.

Dealing with legal and ethical issues

Hospice care is subject to a variety of legal and ethical considerations, and it is the responsibility of hospice case managers to ensure that patients' rights and wishes are respected. This involves navigating complex regulations and guidelines and working closely with patients and their families to help them make difficult decisions about end-of-life care.

One of the challenges of dealing with legal and ethical issues as a hospice case manager is that hospice care involves complex and sensitive issues, such as end-of-life decision-making, pain management, and advanced care planning. This can make it difficult for hospice case managers to navigate these issues, and to ensure that they are acting in accordance with the law and ethical principles. To address this challenge, hospice case managers must be knowledgeable about the legal and ethical considerations that apply to hospice care and must be prepared to consult with legal and ethical experts as needed.

Another challenge is that patients and their families may have different beliefs and values and may have different opinions about what constitutes appropriate care. This can make it difficult for hospice case managers to make decisions that are consistent with the patient's wishes and can lead to conflicts or misunderstandings. To address this challenge, hospice case managers must be able to listen to the needs and preferences of patients and families and work with them to develop a care plan that meets their needs and goals.

In addition, the legal and ethical landscape in the field of hospice care is constantly evolving, and hospice case managers must stay informed about the latest developments and best practices. This may require ongoing education and training and may involve staying up to date with the latest guidelines and regulations. Overall, dealing with legal and ethical issues in hospice care requires a high level of knowledge, sensitivity, and professionalism, and it is an essential part of the role of a hospice case manager.

> "Being a hospice case manager can be challenging, but it is also incredibly rewarding," says Kutselyk. "With the right skills and support, it is possible to overcome these challenges and to provide high-quality care to our patients and their families."

To overcome the challenges faced by hospice case managers, they need to have the right support and resources. Hospice case managers should be part of a strong and supportive hospice care team and should have access to ongoing education and training to help them develop their skills and knowledge.

"Having a strong team and access to resources is essential for the hospice case manager," says Kutselyk. "Without this support, it can be difficult to provide the high-quality care that our patients deserve."

Some specific strategies for overcoming the challenges faced by hospice case managers include:

Collaboration

Collaboration is a crucial aspect of the work of a hospice case manager, and it is essential for ensuring that patients receive the highest quality care possible. In this role, the hospice case manager must work effectively with other members of the hospice care team, including doctors, nurses, social workers, and volunteers, to coordinate and collaborate on the care of their patients. This requires good communication skills, as well as an understanding of the roles and responsibilities of each member of the care team.

In general, healthcare professionals welcome the opportunity to collaborate with their colleagues, as it allows them to share knowledge, expertise, and resources to benefit patients. Collaboration can help to improve the quality of care that patients receive and can lead to better patient outcomes.

For example, when healthcare professionals consult with one another, they may be able to share their different perspectives and expertise and develop a more comprehensive and holistic approach to care. This can be particularly helpful in complex cases, where patients may have multiple medical conditions or may require specialized care.

Collaboration can also help to reduce the risk of errors or mistakes in care, as it allows healthcare professionals to share their knowledge and expertise, and to work together to identify and address potential issues. This can help to ensure that patients receive the most appropriate and effective care possible.

Effective collaboration involves more than just communicating with other team members. It also requires the development of strong working relationships, and the ability to work together as a cohesive team to achieve common goals. This may involve sharing knowledge and expertise, problem-solving together, and supporting one another in the delivery of care.

Pro Tip: Collaboration is a cheat code! Many hands make light work! Teamwork makes the dream work! Etc., etc....

Education and training

Hospice case managers should have access to ongoing education and training to help them develop their skills and knowledge. This may include workshops, conferences, online courses, and other learning opportunities. By staying up to date with the latest developments in hospice care, hospice case managers can provide the best possible care to their patients.

To acquire and maintain the necessary skills and knowledge to provide high-quality care to their patients, hospice case managers need ongoing education and training. There are several different types of education and training that hospice case managers may undergo depending on their specific roles and the needs of their patients. Some examples of education and training for hospice case managers include:

- Clinical training: Hospice case managers may receive training in clinical assessment, symptom and pain management, and other aspects of nursing care. This training may include hands-on experience in a hospice care setting, as well as classroom instruction on topics such as patient care, symptom management, and communication with patients and families.

- Hospice and palliative care education: Hospice case managers may also receive specialized education in hospice and palliative care, including courses on topics such as the principles of hospice care, symptom management, and communication with patients and families. This education may be provided through academic programs, continuing education courses, or on-the-job training programs.

- Certification: Hospice case managers may also choose to become certified in hospice and palliative care through a professional organization such as the National Board for Certification of Hospice and Palliative Nurses. Certification may require passing a written examination and meeting other eligibility requirements, such as having a certain amount of experience in hospice care.

- Ongoing education and professional development: Hospice case managers may also participate in ongoing education and professional development activities to stay up to date on the latest developments in hospice care. This may include attending conferences, workshops, or seminars, reading professional journals, or participating in online learning programs.

Supportive management

Supportive management is crucial for the success of the case manager and care team when providing effective hospice care. In order to provide the best possible care to their patients and their families, it is essential that case managers and their teams feel supported and empowered by their management.

Creating a safe and supportive work environment is a crucial aspect of supportive management. A positive and healthy work culture is essential for the well-being and success of the case manager and care team and can help to ensure that team members are able to provide the best possible care to their patients and their families.

One key aspect of creating a safe and supportive work environment is addressing any issues or conflicts that may arise in a timely and fair manner. This may involve listening to the concerns of team members and working with them to find solutions and taking steps to prevent similar issues from arising in the future. It may also involve providing support and resources to help team members handle challenging or stressful situations and being available to offer guidance and assistance as needed.

Another important aspect of creating a safe and supportive work environment is promoting a healthy work/life balance. This may involve being understanding and flexible when team members need time off or support to handle personal or family matters and helping to create a work culture that values work/life balance and well-being. By promoting a healthy work/life balance, management can help to ensure that team members are able to manage the demands of hospice care while also taking care of their own needs and well-being.

Effective leaders know that the best way to inspire and motivate their team is by leading by example. When management leads from the front, they demonstrate a willingness to work alongside their team and get their hands dirty. This not only fosters a sense of teamwork and collaboration, but also shows that the management team is willing to do whatever it takes to get the job done.

In addition to setting an example through action, supportive management should also be transparent and open in their communication. This means being willing to listen to the ideas and concerns of team members and being open to feedback. By maintaining open lines of communication, management can create a positive and supportive work environment that encourages creativity and innovation.

Overall, leading from the front is an essential aspect of supportive management. It involves setting a good example, being transparent and open in communication, and being willing to listen to the ideas and concerns of team members. By taking this approach, management can help to create a positive and collaborative work culture that inspires and motivates the team to succeed.

Providing clear goals and expectations is an essential aspect of supportive management. By setting clear and specific goals for the case manager and care team, management can help to ensure that team members are working towards shared objectives and that they have a clear sense of purpose and direction. Clear goals can also help to motivate team members and provide a sense of accomplishment when they are achieved.

In addition to setting clear goals, it is also important for management to provide regular feedback to the case manager and care team. This can help to keep team members on track and to ensure that they are meeting the expectations and standards set for them. Regular feedback can also help to identify any areas where team members may need additional support or training and provide an opportunity for management to recognize and reward good work.

Another important aspect of supportive management is helping team members develop their skills and knowledge. This may involve providing training and professional development opportunities and supporting team members in their efforts to learn and grow. By helping team members develop their skills and knowledge, management can help to ensure that the case manager and care team are well-equipped to handle the challenges of hospice care and can provide the highest quality of care to their patients and their families.

Ultimately, supportive management is essential for providing effective hospice care. By providing a safe and supportive environment, and by leading from the front and working with the team towards shared goals, management can help to create a positive and productive work culture and ensure that the case manager and care team are able to provide the best possible care to their patients and their families.

Hospice care can be emotionally demanding for team members, and supportive management is essential in creating a positive work culture.

As hospice case manager Olga Kutselyk RN notes, "Having supportive leadership that respects and guides team members is critical to providing good patient care. By consistently providing constructive and positive guidance, support, and feedback, supportive management can help hospice care teams to work effectively."

Self-care

Hospice case managers should also take care of themselves, both physically and emotionally. This can help them to maintain their own well-being, and to be able to provide the best possible care to their patients. Self-care may include exercise, healthy eating, and other activities that can help to reduce stress and maintain physical and emotional health.

Self-care is the practice of taking care of one's own physical, emotional, and mental health. It is a vital aspect of overall health and well-being and involves activities that help individuals to maintain their health and prevent illness. Self-care can include a wide range of activities, such as exercising regularly, eating a healthy diet, getting enough sleep, managing stress, and engaging in leisure activities. It can also involve seeking professional help when needed, such as seeing a doctor or therapist for physical or mental health concerns.

"Self-care is not selfish. It is essential to our well-being," says licensed clinical social worker Ashley Smith. "When we take care of ourselves, we are better able to take care of others and to handle the challenges that life throws our way."

Some examples of self-care activities include:

- Eating a balanced diet and staying hydrated

- Exercising regularly

- Getting enough sleep

- Managing stress through activities such as meditation, yoga, or journaling

- Engaging in leisure activities that bring joy and relaxation, such as reading, listening to music, or spending time outdoors

- Seeking professional help when needed, such as seeing a doctor for regular check-ups or a therapist for mental health concerns

"Self-care is important because it helps us to stay healthy and to prevent illness," says Smith. "It also allows us to recharge and to feel more balanced and in control of our lives."

The role of a hospice case manager is a crucial one that requires a unique blend of compassion, organization, and collaboration. These professionals are responsible for coordinating and managing the care of patients and their families facing terminal illnesses, ensuring that all their physical, emotional, and spiritual needs are met.

"With the right support and resources, hospice case managers can overcome the challenges of their role and provide high-quality care to their patients," says Kutselyk. "It is important to remember that we are not alone and that we have the support and resources we need to do our best work."

Through effective communication and collaboration with a diverse team of healthcare professionals, hospice case managers can provide comprehensive and coordinated care for patients and their loved ones. They also play a key role in supporting patients and families through the end-of-life journey, offering guidance and support on advance care planning and bereavement.

The hospice case manager is a subject-matter expert on end-of-life care and a valuable resource for patients and families facing the challenges of a terminal illness. Their dedication to providing compassionate care and support makes them an essential member of the healthcare team.

Chapter 3

The Importance of Care Planning and Coordination

As a key member of the hospice care team, the hospice case manager is responsible for developing and implementing a comprehensive care plan for each patient. This care plan is the foundation of the hospice case manager's work and is essential to providing high-quality care to patients who are facing a terminal illness. This care plan serves as a roadmap for the patient's care and is essential to ensuring that all their needs are met in a timely and effective manner. The care plan should be tailored to the individual needs and preferences of the patient and should be developed with input from the patient, their family, and other members of the hospice care team. It should include goals and objectives for the patient's care, as well as a detailed plan for achieving those goals.

The care plan developed by the hospice team will include a plan for managing symptoms and pain, as well as a plan for providing emotional and spiritual support to the patient and their family. It should be reviewed and updated regularly to ensure that it continues to meet the changing needs of the patient. In addition to developing the care plan, the hospice case manager is also responsible for coordinating with other members of the hospice care team to ensure that the plan is implemented effectively. This may involve working closely with doctors, nurses, social workers, and other professionals to provide the best possible care for the patient.

For example, the hospice case manager may work closely with the patient's primary care physician to develop a plan for managing the patient's symptoms and pain. They may also collaborate with nurses and other healthcare professionals to coordinate the delivery of medical care, such as administering medication and providing wound care.

The hospice case manager may also collaborate with social workers and chaplains to provide emotional and spiritual support to the patient and their family. This may involve facilitating access to counseling services or helping the patient and their family navigate the emotional and spiritual challenges that come with facing a terminal illness.

Effective collaboration with other members of the hospice care team requires strong communication skills, the ability to work well in a team environment, and the ability to manage one's own time and workload effectively. It also requires a willingness to listen to the perspectives and expertise of others and to work together to develop solutions to the challenges that may arise in the patient's care.

One key aspect of the hospice case manager's role is to provide families with information about the patient's care, answering their questions and addressing their concerns. This may involve explaining the patient's diagnosis and prognosis, providing information about treatment options, and discussing the goals and objectives of the care plan. The hospice case manager should also be available to provide ongoing support and guidance to the patient and their family as needed.

In addition to providing information and support, the hospice case manager should also involve the patient and their family in decision-making. This may involve discussing the patient's treatment options and preferences with them and ensuring that their rights and preferences are respected. The hospice case manager will work closely with the patient and their family to develop a plan for managing the patient's symptoms and pain, as well as a plan for providing emotional and spiritual support.

Coordinating care and communication can be challenging, especially in a complex healthcare system. The hospice case manager should have strong organizational skills and should be able to manage their own time and workload effectively. They should also have access to resources and support to help them overcome any challenges they may face.

Some specific benefits of care planning and coordination in hospice care include:

- Improved patient outcomes: By providing a comprehensive and individualized care plan, the hospice case manager can help to improve patient outcomes. This may include reducing symptoms and pain, improving quality of life, and providing emotional and spiritual support.

- Enhanced communication: By coordinating with other members of the hospice care team, and by communicating regularly with the patient and their family, the hospice case manager can help to enhance communication and collaboration. This can help to ensure that patients receive timely and appropriate care and can help to avoid misunderstandings and miscommunications.

- Increased patient satisfaction: By involving the patient and their family in care planning and decision-making, the hospice case manager can help to increase patient satisfaction. This may include ensuring that patients' rights and preferences are respected and providing them with the information and support they need to make informed decisions about their care.

- Greater efficiency: By coordinating care and communication, the hospice case manager can help to increase the efficiency of the hospice care team. This may include reducing unnecessary tests and procedures and avoiding duplication of efforts. By working efficiently, the hospice case manager can help to ensure that patients receive the care they need in a timely and effective manner.

In addition to the benefits of care planning and coordination, there are also some potential challenges and barriers that the hospice case manager may face in their work. These challenges can vary depending on the setting and the individual needs of the patient, but some common challenges include:

- Limited time and resources: Developing and implementing a comprehensive care plan can be time-consuming and resource-intensive. Hospice case managers may face challenges in managing their workload, and in accessing the resources they need to provide high-quality care.

- Communication barriers: Coordinating care and communication can be challenging, especially in a complex healthcare system. Hospice case managers may face barriers in communicating with other members of the hospice care team, and in ensuring that patients and their families receive the information and support they need.

- Legal and ethical considerations: Hospice care is subject to a variety of legal and ethical considerations, and hospice case managers must be aware of these issues. They may face challenges in navigating complex regulations and guidelines, and in ensuring that patients' rights and wishes are respected.

- Patient and family dynamics: The hospice case manager may also face challenges in managing the dynamics of the patient's family and other caregivers. This may include dealing with conflicts, providing support, and facilitating communication among family members.

The following are two example care plans with some potential interventions. The actual formatting of the care plan, as well as specific goals and interventions, may be set by the hospice provider. Additionally, the care plan used will likely have more detailed and patient-specific goals and interventions. The case manager will work within the guidelines set by the hospice provider for how the information is formatted.

Note that there is a *terminal diagnosis* as well as *nursing diagnoses*. A terminal diagnosis is a determination made by a healthcare provider, such as a doctor, of the condition or disease a patient is suffering from based on an evaluation of their symptoms and medical history. The terminal diagnosis is usually a medical diagnosis. A nursing diagnosis is a determination made by a nurse of the patient's health issues or needs based on an evaluation of their physical, emotional, and spiritual well-being.

Terminal diagnoses are made by doctors and are based on the results of medical tests, such as blood tests or imaging studies, as well as the patient's symptoms, medical history, and prognosis. They are used to determine the appropriate course of treatment for the patient's medical condition.

Nursing diagnoses, on the other hand, are made by nurses and are based on a comprehensive assessment of the patient's physical, emotional, and spiritual well-being. They are used to identify the patient's health issues or needs and to guide the development of a nursing care plan. Nursing diagnoses may be related to medical diagnoses, but they go beyond the medical condition and focus on the patient's overall health and well-being.

Patient: 72-year-old male with lung cancer, pain, dyspnea

Terminal Diagnosis: Stage IV lung cancer

Nursing Diagnosis: Pain related to cancer and treatment

Problems:
The patient is experiencing chronic pain related to their cancer and treatment.

Goals:
The patient will report a reduction in pain from an 8 to a 4 on a scale of 0-10 within 2 weeks.

Interventions:
- Administer pain medication according to the prescribed schedule
- Educate the patient and their family about pain management techniques, such as relaxation techniques and proper positioning, to supplement pharmacological treatment

Nursing Diagn: Shortness of breath related to cancer and treatment

Problems:
- The patient is experiencing shortness of breath related to their cancer and treatment.

Goals:
- The patient will be able to breathe comfortably and maintain oxygen saturation within normal limits.

Interventions:
- Assist the patient with deep breathing and coughing techniques to manage shortness of breath
- Provide oxygen therapy as prescribed

Nursing Diagnosis: Risk for impaired skin integrity related to immobility

Problems:
- The patient is at risk for pressure ulcers due to immobility.

Goals:
- The patient will maintain skin integrity and prevent pressure ulcers.

Interventions:
- Perform skin assessments regularly and implement preventive measures, such as turning and repositioning, to maintain skin integrity
- Change dressings and provide wound care as needed

Nursing Diagnosis: Risk for malnutrition related to difficulty with eating and drinking

Problems:
- The patient is at risk for malnutrition due to difficulty with eating and drinking.

Goals:
- The patient will maintain nutrition and hydration status.

Interventions:
- Encourage the patient to consume a well-balanced diet and offer assistance with eating and drinking as needed

- Provide nutrition and hydration through oral, enteral, or parenteral routes as needed

Nursing Diagn: Spiritual distress related to terminal illness

Problems:
- The patient is experiencing spiritual distress related to their terminal illness.

Goals:
- The patient will experience a sense of peace and closure as they near the end of life.

Interventions:
- Offer emotional and spiritual support to the patient and their family through one-on-one counseling and support groups
- Facilitate access to chaplain services as requested
- Encourage the patient and their family to express their feelings and discuss their concerns
- Assist the patient in completing advanced care planning documents, such as a living will and durable power of attorney for healthcare
- Encourage the patient to engage in activities that bring meaning and purpose to their life, such as spending time with loved ones or participating in hobbies

Coordination of Care:
- Coordinate with the patient's primary care physician and other members of the hospice care team to ensure that their medical needs are met
- Communicate with the patient and their family regularly to keep them informed about their care and to address any concerns they may have
- Work with the patient and their family to develop a plan for managing symptoms and pain, as well as a plan for providing emotional and spiritual support
- Monitor the patient's nutrition and hydration status and implement interventions as needed.

Patient: 84-year-old male patient ALS, chronic pain, emphysema, GERD, paralysis, depression, and hypertension

Terminal Diagnosis: ALS

Nursing Diagnosis: Acute pain related to ALS, emphysema, and GERD.

Problems:
- Patient is experiencing chronic pain and discomfort that affects their ability to perform activities of daily living.
- Patient is unable to communicate their pain and discomfort effectively due to paralysis.

Goals:
- The patient will report a reduction in pain from an 7 to a 4 on a scale of 0-10 within 2 weeks.
- The patient will be able to participate in activities of daily living with minimal assistance within 4 weeks.
- The patient will be able to communicate their pain effectively within 2 weeks.

Interventions:
- Assess the patient's pain level and location daily, and document in the patient's chart.
- Administer prescribed pain medication as ordered and reassess pain level after medication administration.
- Implement non-pharmacologic pain management techniques such as relaxation techniques and positioning for comfort.
- Refer the patient to physical therapy to assist with maintaining mobility and function.
- Collaborate with the interdisciplinary team to evaluate the patient's need for equipment such as a hospital bed and Hoyer lift to assist with mobility.
- Utilize alternative methods of communication such as eye movements or other non-verbal cues to assess and manage the patient's pain effectively.

Nursing Diagn: Depression related to diagnosis of ALS and loss of function

Problems:
- Patient is experiencing feelings of hopelessness and helplessness due to the diagnosis of ALS and the associated loss of function.
- Patient is experiencing a lack of interest in activities and a decreased ability to participate in enjoyable activities.

Goals:
- The patient will report an improvement in mood and an increase in positive affect within 2 weeks.
- The patient will be able to participate in enjoyable activities with minimal assistance within 4 weeks.
- The patient will have improved communication and involvement with family and friends.

Interventions:
- Assess the patient's mood and affect daily, and document in the patient's chart.
- Provide emotional support and validation to the patient and their family.
- Encourage the patient to participate in activities they enjoy, such as reading or listening to music.
- Refer the patient to a counselor or social worker for further emotional support.
- Collaborate with the interdisciplinary team to provide bereavement support for the patient and their family.
- Encourage the patient to communicate their feelings and thoughts to their family and friends.
- Encourage the patient to involve family and friends in their care plan.

Nursing Diagnosis: Risk for complications related to hypertension

Problems:
- Patient has hypertension and is at risk for complications related to hypertension such as stroke, heart attack, and kidney damage.
- Patient lacks knowledge about hypertension and its management.

Goals:
- The patient will have blood pressure within normal limits (less than 140/90 mm Hg) within 2 weeks.
- The patient will demonstrate understanding of the importance of maintaining a healthy diet and exercise regimen.
- The patient will report improved quality of life.

Interventions:
- Assess the patient's blood pressure daily and document in the patient's chart.
- Administer prescribed hypertension medication as ordered.

- Collaborate with the interdisciplinary team to provide education on hypertension and the importance of maintaining a healthy diet and exercise regimen.
- Encourage the patient to adhere to a low-salt, low-fat diet and provide resources for healthy meal planning.
- Monitor the patient's blood pressure regularly and collaborate with the physician to adjust medication as needed.
- Encourage the patient to adhere to a regular follow-up schedule with their primary care provider to monitor hypertension control.
- Encourage the patient to maintain a healthy lifestyle by reducing stress, avoid smoking and limit alcohol intake.
- Encourage the patient to take an active role in their care and communicate any concerns or questions to the healthcare team.
- Collaborate with the patient's primary care provider to ensure continuity of care and appropriate follow-up.

The importance of care planning and coordination in hospice care cannot be overstated. By developing a comprehensive and individualized care plan, collaborating with other members of the hospice care team, and coordinating and communicating with families, the hospice case manager plays a vital role in ensuring that patients receive the high-quality care they deserve.

Chapter 4

Clinical Assessment and Symptom Management

Hospice case managers have the opportunity to work with patients during a time of great reflection and introspection. Your role is to assess and address their physical, emotional, and spiritual needs in order to provide the best possible end-of-life care. These assessments involve having meaningful conversations with patients about their lives, experiences, and feelings. These conversations often involve sharing stories and memories and can be deeply personal and emotional for both the patient and the case manager.

One of the most challenging aspects of working in hospice care is dealing with the knowledge that our patients are facing the end of their lives. This can be particularly distressing for some patients with illnesses such as cancer who may not feel very ill until the final stages of their disease. As hospice professionals, it is our job to provide support and comfort to these patients and to help them find resolution and closure as they come to terms with their mortality.

Working in hospice care is deeply rewarding but also a weighty responsibility. It requires compassion, empathy, and a commitment to providing the best possible care to our patients. It is not a field to be entered into lightly, and I believe it is important for those working in this field to approach their work with the utmost care and respect for the patients and families they serve.

As a hospice case manager, one of your primary responsibilities is to conduct thorough assessments of your patients to identify and manage their symptoms and pain. This is essential to provide high-quality care and ensure that patients are as comfortable as possible in their final days. This chapter goes over some of the most common types of assessments a hospice case manager will perform as well as symptom management and treatment options.

When conducting an assessment, the nurse must always take a holistic approach that considers the patient's physical, emotional, and spiritual needs. This will involve gathering information from the patient, their family, and other members of the hospice care team, as well as conducting a physical examination.

One of the key components of a clinical assessment is identifying and managing symptoms and pain. This may include administering medications to control pain, providing comfort measures such as massage or heat therapy, and collaborating with other members of the care team to develop a comprehensive plan for symptom management. In addition, a hospice nurse will provide emotional and spiritual support to patients and their families. This may involve listening to their concerns and fears, offering words of comfort and reassurance, and connecting them with chaplains or other spiritual care providers.

A hospice nurse will use a variety of assessments when completing a thorough hospice assessment. These may include a physical assessment, which involves evaluating the patient's vital signs, body systems, and overall physical health. The nurse may also perform a cognitive assessment, which involves evaluating the patient's mental status and ability to understand and make decisions about their care. In addition, the nurse may conduct a psychosocial assessment, which involves evaluating the patient's social and emotional well-being, including their relationships and support system. The nurse may also assess the patient's spiritual well-being, including their beliefs, values, and end-of-life wishes. By using these different types of assessments, the hospice nurse gains a comprehensive understanding of the patient's overall health and well-being and develops a care plan that addresses their physical, mental, emotional, and spiritual needs.

Case study: The Hospice Nurse Case Manager, Sarah, was assigned to the case of Mrs. Alice Nesbitt. Mrs. Nesbitt was an 85-year-old widow who had recently lost her husband of 60 years, Tom, to an illness. Sarah was introduced to Mrs. Nesbitt by the community liaison, Theresa, who had been contacted by Mrs. Nesbitt's daughter and Power of Attorney, Janice, after she found her mother on the floor of her kitchen, blue in the face.

Following several diagnostic tests, it was determined by her primary care physician Dr. Harris that Mrs. Nesbitt's COPD and CHF had worsened, and her prognosis was 6 months or less. Mrs. Nesbitt expressed her wishes to remain comfortable in her final days in lieu of aggressive and invasive treatment. Dr. Harris recommended that she be evaluated for hospice care.

Theresa and Sarah explained the hospice care program and its interdisciplinary approach to Mrs. Nesbitt and her daughter, including the different members of the hospice care team and the services they provide. Following an emotional conversation in which Sarah and Theresa were able to provide some emotional and spiritual support, Mrs. Nesbitt signed the admission paperwork acknowledging that she fully understood her choice and that she consented to treatment by the hospice provider.

Mrs. Nesbitt was admitted to hospice services and the hospice team, led by Sarah, developed a care plan to address her physical, emotional, and spiritual needs.

Conducting a Hospice Nurse Clinical Assessment

A hospice nurse clinical assessment is a comprehensive evaluation of the patient's physical, emotional, and social needs. This assessment is typically performed at the beginning of the hospice care process and is updated on a regular basis to reflect any changes in the patient's condition.

By completing a clinical assessment with every visit, the hospice nurse can gather accurate and up-to-date information about the patient's condition. This can help the nurse to identify any changes or concerns that may need to be addressed. The clinical assessment is also used to develop a plan of care that is tailored to the patient's individual needs. By completing a clinical assessment with every visit, the hospice nurse can ensure that the plan of care remains current and appropriate for the patient's changing needs.

A clinical assessment can also help the hospice nurse to identify potential issues early on and take action to address them before they become more serious. This can be especially important in the hospice setting, where the focus is on providing symptom relief and end-of-life support.

Additionally, a clinical assessment can help the hospice nurse identify any symptoms that the patient may be experiencing and take steps to improve the patient's comfort and quality of life. This may involve administering medications to manage pain or discomfort or providing emotional support to the patient and their family.

Finally, a clinical assessment can provide the hospice nurse with an opportunity to connect with the patient and their family, offering support and guidance as needed. This can be especially imperative during the end-of-life process, as it can help to alleviate some of the stress and uncertainty that the patient and their family may be experiencing.

- Begin the assessment by introducing yourself and explaining the purpose of the assessment to the patient. Gather information from the patient, their family, and other members of the hospice care team. This may include medical records, previous assessments, and information about the patient's physical, emotional, and spiritual needs.

- Ask for the patient's permission to perform the assessment and reassure them that they can stop the assessment at any time if they feel uncomfortable.

- Conduct a physical examination, including measurements such as pulse, blood pressure, respiratory rate, and temperature. Observe the patient for any signs of discomfort or distress and document your findings.

- Identify any symptoms or concerns, such as pain, shortness of breath, fatigue, or constipation. Ask the patient about their level of pain and assess their ability to perform activities of daily living.

- Develop a plan for managing the patient's symptoms and pain, in collaboration with other members of the care team. This may include administering medications, providing comfort measures, or referring the patient to other specialists.

- Provide emotional and spiritual support to the patient and their family. This may involve listening to their concerns and fears, offering words of comfort, and connecting them with chaplains or other spiritual care providers.

- Document the assessment thoroughly and accurately, including any changes in the patient's condition, interventions, and follow-up plans.

- Follow up with the patient and their family to monitor their progress and adjust the care plan as needed. Continue to provide support and assistance to help the patient and their family through the end-of-life journey.

Case study: Sarah, the hospice case manager, began her assessment of Mrs. Nesbitt by introducing herself and explaining the purpose of the assessment. Even though Sarah may have made several prior visits, Mrs. Nesbitt has mild dementia and may not reveal that she doesn't recall who Sarah is. Sarah makes her patient feel more comfortable by curating a safe place for her assessment to take place prior to every visit. For this reason, it is vitally important that Sarah calls before her visit to help prepare Mrs. Nesbitt and her daughter, who is Power of Attorney.

When Sarah arrived for her visit, she gathered information from Mrs. Nesbitt and her daughter Janice, including medical records, previous assessments, and information about the patient's physical, emotional, and spiritual needs.

Sarah asked for Mrs. Nesbitt's permission to perform the assessment and reassured her that she can stop the assessment at any time if she feels uncomfortable. She conducted a physical examination, including measurements such as pulse, blood pressure, respiratory rate, and temperature, and observed Mrs. Nesbitt for any signs of discomfort or distress and documented her findings.

Sarah identified any symptoms or concerns, such as pain, shortness of breath, fatigue, or constipation. She asked Mrs. Nesbitt about her level of pain and assessed her ability to perform activities of daily living. Sarah also developed a plan for managing Mrs. Nesbitt's symptoms and pain, in collaboration with other members of the care team. This included administering medications, providing comfort measures, and referring the patient to other specialists.

Sarah provided emotional and spiritual support to Mrs. Nesbitt and her family. This involved listening to their concerns and fears, offering words of comfort, and connecting them with the hospice chaplain. Sarah then documented the assessment thoroughly and accurately, including any changes in the patient's condition, interventions, and follow-up plans.

The following are some examples of common assessments the hospice nurse will complete with each visit. Each hospice provider will have specific guidance for the hospice nurse case manager to follow when completing assessments. It is the case manager's responsibility to follow their hospice agency's policies and applicable laws regarding documentation, as well as perform the necessary assessments needed to collect enough data to create a comprehensive care plan.

Performing a Head-to-Toe Physical Assessment

The hospice nurse will perform a physical evaluation with every visit to assess the patient's physical condition and identify any changes or concerns. This evaluation is a significant part of the hospice care process, as it helps the nurse to understand the patient's needs and develop a plan of care that is tailored to their individual needs.

- Begin the assessment at the patient's head, observing their face for any signs of distress or discomfort. Ask the patient about their vision, hearing, and ability to speak. Check the patient's head and scalp for any abnormalities, such as lumps, bumps, or bruises.

- Move down to the patient's neck and shoulders, checking for any tenderness or stiffness. Observe the patient's neck for any swelling or asymmetry. Check the patient's range of motion in their neck and shoulders and note any limitations or pain.

- Proceed to the patient's chest and lungs, observing the patient's breathing pattern and listening to their breath sounds with a stethoscope. Ask the patient about any coughing or shortness of breath, and check for any chest pain or discomfort.

- Continue the assessment by examining the patient's abdomen, checking for any tenderness, swelling, or masses. Ask the patient about their bowel movements, appetite, and any nausea or vomiting.

- Move to the patient's arms and hands, checking for any swelling, tenderness, or deformities. Observe the patient's grip strength and range of motion in their arms and hands, and check for any swelling or discoloration in the wrists and fingers.

- Proceed to the patient's legs and feet, checking for any swelling, tenderness, or deformities. Observe the patient's gait and balance, and check for any swelling or discoloration in the ankles and toes.

Performing a Thorough Skin Check on a Hospice Patient

The hospice nurse performs a skin evaluation with every visit to assess the patient's skin condition and identify any changes or concerns. This evaluation is an important part of the hospice care process, as the skin is often one of the first areas to show signs of changes in the patient's health.

By performing a skin evaluation on a regular basis, the hospice nurse can identify potential skin issues early on and take action to address them before they become more serious. The skin is also a good indicator of the patient's overall health, and changes in the skin can be a sign of underlying issues. By performing a skin evaluation, the hospice nurse can get a better understanding of the patient's health and identify any potential problems that may need to be addressed.

A skin evaluation can also help the hospice nurse to identify any symptoms that the patient may be experiencing, such as itching or pain. By addressing these symptoms, the nurse can help to improve the patient's comfort and quality of life.

In terms of the skin in dying patients, it is common for the skin to undergo changes as the patient approaches the end of life. These changes can include thinning of the skin, changes in color, dryness, bruising or discoloration, and temperature changes. The hospice nurse needs to be aware of these changes and take steps to address any symptoms that may be causing the patient discomfort. This may involve using moisturizers to prevent dryness, administering medications to manage pain or itching, and providing emotional support to the patient and their family.

- Begin the skin check at the patient's head, using a bright light to carefully examine their face, scalp, and neck. Look for any signs of redness, swelling, or irritation, and note any areas of concern.

- Proceed to the patient's chest and upper body, using the light to carefully examine their chest, back, and arms. Look for any signs of redness, swelling, or irritation, and note any areas of concern.

- Continue the skin check by examining the patient's lower body, including the abdomen, groin, thighs, and legs. Use the light to carefully examine these areas, looking for any signs of redness, swelling, or irritation, and note any areas of concern.

- Pay special attention to any areas of the patient's skin that are prone to pressure wounds, such as the heels, ankles, and elbows. Carefully examine these areas, looking for any signs of redness, swelling, or irritation, and note any areas of concern.
- If you identify any areas of concern during the skin check, document these findings thoroughly and accurately. Follow up with the patient and the care team to develop a plan for managing any skin issues, including the prevention and treatment of pressure wounds.

Pressure wounds, also known as pressure ulcers or bedsores, are areas of damage to the skin and underlying tissue that occur as a result of prolonged pressure on the skin. They are common in hospice patients, particularly those who are bedridden or have limited mobility.

Pressure wounds occur when the skin and underlying tissue are subjected to prolonged pressure, which disrupts the blood flow to the affected area. This can cause the skin and tissue to break down and become damaged. Pressure wounds are typically found on bony areas of the body, such as the heels, ankles, and hips, where the skin is thin and there is less padding to protect the tissue from the pressure.

There are several factors that can increase the risk of pressure wounds in hospice patients. These include advanced age, impaired mobility, incontinence, malnutrition, and certain medical conditions, such as diabetes or peripheral vascular disease. In hospice patients, pressure wounds can be particularly challenging to identify and treat due to the nature of the patient's terminal illness and the focus on comfort and symptom management rather than cure.

One of the main challenges in identifying and treating pressure wounds in hospice patients is the fact that they may not exhibit the usual symptoms, such as pain or redness. This can make it difficult for healthcare providers to detect the presence of a pressure wound in its early stages. In addition, hospice patients may be unable to report symptoms due to their advanced illness or the use of pain medication, which can mask the symptoms of a pressure wound.

Treatment of pressure wounds in hospice patients can be challenging due to the patient's terminal illness and the focus on comfort and symptom management. The main goal of treatment is to prevent the pressure wound from worsening and to promote healing, if possible. This may involve relieving pressure on the affected area, cleaning and dressing the wound, and providing nutrition and hydration to support the healing process. In some cases, surgical intervention may be necessary to remove dead tissue or to promote healing.

To identify pressure sores, follow these steps:

- Look for areas of red, painful, or swollen skin, especially on bony prominences such as the heels, ankles, tailbone, and lower back.

- Check for blisters, open wounds, or pus-like drainage.

- Gently press on the skin around the sore. If the skin does not quickly return to its normal shape or color, it may be a pressure sore.

- Check for areas of the skin that feel cool to the touch or have a different temperature than the surrounding skin.

- Pay attention to any changes in the size or appearance of the sore.

If a hospice nurse suspects that a patient has a pressure ulcer, they should take the following steps:

- Conduct a thorough assessment of the wound, including its location, size, depth, and appearance.

- Document the findings of the assessment in the patient's medical record.

- Clean the wound using a sterile saline solution and gentle cleansing techniques.

- Cover the wound with a sterile, moisture-absorbing dressing to promote healing and prevent infection.

- Monitor the wound for any changes in size, appearance, or odor.

- Keep the patient's skin clean and dry.

- Reposition the patient every two hours or as needed to prevent pressure on any one area of the skin.

- Use pillows or foam wedges to support the patient in a comfortable position.

- Keep the patient's nutrition and hydration levels up to prevent dry, thin skin.

- Avoid rubbing or massaging the skin, as this can cause irritation.

- Use a special mattress or cushion designed to relieve pressure on the skin.

In addition to the steps above, hospice nurses may also recommend the following treatments for pressure ulcers:

- Medications to reduce pain and inflammation

- Specialized dressings to promote healing and prevent infection

- Nutritional support to promote wound healing and prevent malnutrition

- Off-loading devices to relieve pressure on the affected area

- Physical therapy to improve circulation and prevent further pressure ulcers

- Referral to a home health provider for advanced wound care

Hospice nurses must accurately stage pressure ulcers to determine the appropriate treatment plan. The National Pressure Ulcer Advisory Panel (NPUAP) has developed a staging system for pressure ulcers that is widely used in the medical community. The stages of pressure ulcers are as follows:

Stage 1: A reddened area of skin that does not blanch (turn pale) when pressed. There is no open wound or break in the skin. Stage 1 pressure wounds are superficial and do not extend past the epidermis, or outer layer of the skin. They may appear red and swollen and may be painful to the touch.

To stage a stage 1 pressure wound, the hospice nurse will assess the wound using the following criteria:

- Size: The size of the wound is measured in inches or centimeters.

- Depth: The depth of the wound is determined by how deep the wound extends into the skin. In a stage 1 pressure wound, the depth is limited to the epidermis.

- Tissue involvement: The hospice nurse will assess the condition of the surrounding tissue, including the presence of inflammation or infection.

- Exudate: The hospice nurse will assess the amount and type of drainage from the wound.

Treatment for a stage 1 pressure wound may include cleaning the wound and applying a dressing to protect the area and promote healing. It may also involve relieving pressure on the affected area to prevent further breakdown of the skin.

Stage 2: A shallow open wound with a reddened area of skin around it. The wound may be filled with clear or yellow fluid. Stage 2 pressure wounds are deeper than stage 1 wounds and extend into the dermis or the inner layer of the skin. They may appear red and swollen and may be painful to the touch. There may also be some drainage or exudate present.

To stage a stage 2 pressure wound, the hospice nurse will assess the wound using the same criteria as a stage 1 wound: size, depth, tissue involvement, and exudate. In addition to these criteria, the hospice nurse will also consider the presence of *undermining* and *tunneling*, which are when the wound extends under the skin and forms small passages or channels.

Treatment for a stage 2 pressure wound may include cleaning the wound, removing any dead or damaged tissue, and applying a dressing to protect the area and promote healing. It may also involve relieving pressure on the affected area to prevent further breakdown of the skin. In some cases, surgery may be necessary to remove dead or damaged tissue and promote healing.

Stage 3: A deeper wound with a crater-like appearance. The wound may extend into the underlying tissue and may contain dead tissue. Stage 3 pressure wounds are deeper than stage 1 and stage 2 wounds and extend into the subcutaneous tissue, which is the layer of fat and connective tissue underneath the skin. They may appear red and swollen and may be painful to the touch. There may also be a significant amount of drainage or exudate present.

To stage a stage 3 pressure wound, the hospice nurse will assess the wound using the same criteria as stage 1 and stage 2 wounds: size, depth, tissue involvement, and exudate. In addition to these criteria, the healthcare professional will also consider the presence of undermining and tunneling, which are when the wound extends under the skin and forms small passages or channels.

Treatment for a stage 3 pressure wound may include cleaning the wound, removing any dead or damaged tissue, and applying a dressing to protect the area and promote healing. It may also involve relieving pressure on the affected area to prevent further breakdown of the skin. In some cases, surgery may be necessary to remove dead or damaged tissue and promote healing. Stage 3 pressure wounds often take longer to heal than stage 1 or stage 2 wounds and may require ongoing treatment and wound care.

Stage 4: The most severe stage of a pressure ulcer, in which the wound extends into the muscle and bone and may be infected. Stage 4 pressure wounds are the most severe type of pressure wound and extend into the muscle and bone. They may appear red and swollen and may be painful to the touch. There may also be a significant amount of drainage or exudate present.

To stage a stage 4 pressure wound, the hospice nurse will assess the wound using the same criteria as stage 1, stage 2, and stage 3 wounds: size, depth, tissue involvement, and exudate. In addition to these criteria, the hospice nurse will also consider the presence of undermining and tunneling, which are when the wound extends under the skin and forms small passages or channels.

Treatment for a stage 4 pressure wound may include cleaning the wound, removing any dead or damaged tissue, and applying a dressing to protect the area and promote healing. It may also involve relieving pressure on the affected area to prevent further breakdown of the skin. In some cases, surgery may be necessary to remove dead or damaged tissue and promote healing. Stage 4 pressure wounds often take longer to heal than stage 1, stage 2, or stage 3 wounds, and may require ongoing treatment and wound care.

Deep tissue injuries (DTI) are a type of pressure sore that occurs when damage to the skin and underlying tissue is not immediately visible. DTIs often develop in areas of the body that are subjected to prolonged pressure and are most common in people who are bedridden or have limited mobility, such as hospice patients.

DTI's are not the same as Stage 1 pressure wounds. Symptoms of a DTI may include a patch of skin that is dark purple or maroon in color, swelling, and pain. The area may also feel firm or boggy to the touch. DTIs can progress rapidly and can become serious, potentially life-threatening infections if left untreated.

Stage 1 pressure wounds, on the other hand, are the least severe type of pressure sore. They typically appear as a reddened area of skin that does not blanch (turn pale) when pressure is applied. Stage 1 pressure wounds may be painful, but they do not usually involve broken skin or visible tissue damage.

To prevent DTIs in hospice patients, it is important to follow the same preventative measures used to prevent other types of pressure sores, such as regularly repositioning the patient, keeping the skin clean and dry, and using special mattresses or cushions to relieve pressure on the skin. It is also important to monitor the patient for any changes in skin color or texture and to notify a healthcare professional if a DTI is suspected.

If a DTI is present, treatment will typically involve cleaning and dressing the wound, providing pain medication, and repositioning the patient to prevent further pressure on the affected area. It is also important to address any underlying medical conditions that may be contributing to the development of the DTI, such as pressure, nutritional compromise, and dehydration.

A *Kennedy terminal ulcer* is a deep, painful wound that sometimes develops in patients who are dying or near the end of life. These ulcers are typically found on the sacrum, lower legs, or ankles and are characterized by necrosis (death of tissue) and sloughing (shedding or separation) of the skin and underlying tissues. They may also have a foul odor due to the presence of necrotic tissue and/or infection.

Kennedy terminal ulcers are often caused by a combination of factors, including poor circulation, immobility, and malnutrition. They can also be the result of underlying medical conditions such as diabetes, peripheral arterial disease, or venous insufficiency.

The management of Kennedy terminal ulcers typically involves a combination of wound care and pain management. This may involve cleaning and dressing the ulcer, using specialized wound care products to promote healing and prevent infection, and administering pain medications as needed. The hospice nurse must address any underlying issues that may be contributing to the development of the ulcer, such as poor circulation or malnutrition, to optimize the patient's comfort and improve the chances of healing.

The hospice nurse must be able to recognize the signs and symptoms of pressure ulcers and take immediate and appropriate action to prevent, treat, and manage these wounds. This may include conducting thorough assessments, providing appropriate wound care, and recommending specialized treatments. By following best practices and providing high-quality care, hospice nurses can help their patients heal from pressure ulcers and maintain their quality of life.

Assessing For and Treating Dehydration

Dehydration is a common concern in hospice patients and can have significant impacts on their health and quality of life. It occurs when the body lacks sufficient fluids to function properly and can result in symptoms such as dry mouth, thirst, fatigue, dizziness, and dark urine. In severe cases, dehydration can lead to serious complications, such as kidney damage, confusion, and falls.

Hospice patients are at increased risk of dehydration due to a variety of factors, including advanced age, decreased mobility, and certain medical conditions, such as diabetes or kidney disease. In addition, hospice patients may be more prone to dehydration due to the side effects of their medications or the presence of a terminal illness that affects their ability to consume fluids.

The hospice nurse plays a crucial role in identifying and treating dehydration in hospice patients. They should assess the patient's hydration status regularly and look for signs of dehydration, such as dry mouth, dark urine, and fatigue. If the nurse suspects that the patient is dehydrated, they should take steps to rehydrate the patient and prevent further dehydration.

Treatment of dehydration in hospice patients may involve increasing fluid intake, either through oral fluids or intravenous fluids, as well as adjusting the patient's medications or other interventions as needed. The hospice nurse should work closely with the patient and their family to identify strategies to increase fluid intake and to monitor the patient's response to treatment.

The hospice nurse must identify and treat dehydration in patients in a timely manner to prevent complications and to improve the patient's quality of life. Dehydration can significantly impact the patient's comfort and ability to function, and prompt treatment can help to alleviate these symptoms and improve the patient's overall well-being.

To assess a patient for dehydration, the hospice nurse should look for the following signs and symptoms:

- Elevated body temperature: Dehydration can cause the body to produce more heat, leading to an elevated body temperature.

- Low blood pressure: Dehydration can cause the volume of blood in the body to drop, leading to low blood pressure.

- Rapid pulse: When the body is dehydrated, the heart has to work harder to pump blood, leading to a rapid pulse.

- Dry mouth and skin: Dehydration can cause the mouth and skin to become dry, as the body is not producing enough saliva and sweat.

- Fatigue and weakness: Dehydration can cause a person to feel tired and weak, as the body is not getting enough fluids to function properly.

- Decreased urine output or dark-colored urine

- Sunken eyes

If a patient exhibits any of these signs or symptoms, the hospice nurse should take steps to treat the dehydration. This may involve providing the patient with fluids, either orally or, less commonly, through an intravenous (IV) line. The type and amount of fluids will depend on the severity of the dehydration and the patient's overall health status.

In pre-hospice settings, intravenous (IV) hydration can be a useful tool in helping to manage symptoms and improve the comfort of the dying patient. Some patients and family members may request that dehydration be treated with IV hydration. However, there are potential dangers associated with IV hydration, particularly in advanced stages of illness.

One potential danger of IV hydration is the risk of fluid overload, which can occur when too much fluid is administered too quickly. This can lead to an accumulation of fluid in the body's tissues, which can cause swelling, shortness of breath, and other symptoms. In severe cases, fluid overload can be life-threatening.

Fluid overload can occur when too much fluid is retained in the body's tissues, causing a build-up of excess fluid in the lungs, heart, and other organs. This can lead to swelling (edema), shortness of breath, and other symptoms. In severe cases, fluid overload can cause the heart to fail, resulting in serious complications or death.

The hospice nurse should identify and address any underlying causes of dehydration. This may include illness, diarrhea, vomiting, or medications that can cause dehydration. The hospice nurse should work with the patient and their healthcare team to develop a plan to address these underlying causes and prevent future episodes of dehydration.

In addition to providing fluids, the hospice nurse can also help prevent dehydration by encouraging the patient to drink plenty of fluids and eat foods that are high in water content, such as fruits and vegetables. The hospice nurse should also monitor the patient's fluid intake and output and make any necessary adjustments to the treatment plan.

Overall, the goal of treating dehydration in hospice patients is to restore the body's fluid balance and prevent complications such as electrolyte imbalances, kidney damage, and other health problems. By regularly assessing patients for signs of dehydration and providing appropriate treatment, the hospice nurse can help improve the patient's quality of life and prevent further complications from developing.

Case study: During a visit to Mrs. Nesbitt, Sarah, the hospice nurse, assessed her patient and identified that she was experiencing symptoms of dehydration. Mrs. Nesbitt reported that she had not been drinking many fluids due to feeling tired and not wanting to get up to refill her cup. Sarah's assessment revealed that Mrs. Nesbitt had vital signs outside of her normal baseline parameters, including low blood pressure, rapid pulse, decreased urine output with dark-colored urine, and fatigue and weakness.

Mrs. Nesbitt's daughter, Janice, was present during the visit and expressed her desire to have her mother transported to the hospital for IV hydration. Sarah calmly provided emotional support to both Janice and Mrs. Nesbitt and compassionately explained the potential risks of IV hydration in a dying patient, particularly in those with CHF, as it may cause fluid overload which could lead to a heart attack or death. Sarah informed both Janice and Mrs. Nesbitt that seeking treatment at the hospital was their choice, but that it would result in Mrs. Nesbitt being revoked from hospice services during her hospital stay. However, it was also explained that she could be re-evaluated for hospice services once she returned home if she wished to consider hospice care in lieu of curative treatment.

To address the dehydration symptoms, Sarah suggested that every morning Janice fill a pitcher of water and place it on the coffee table in the living room and place several bottles of water around the house so that Mrs. Nesbitt had water nearby wherever she was in her home. Janice also suggested placing a glass next to every sink, so that Mrs. Nesbitt could fill it with water and take a drink. Sarah thanked Janice for participating in the plan of care and Mrs. Nesbitt agreed to these interventions. On Sarah's next visit, she found that Mrs. Nesbitt was showing fewer symptoms of dehydration and appeared to have more energy. Janice also reported that her mother had even been less forgetful lately.

Assessing For and Treating Bowel Complications

The hospice nurse will regularly assess the patient for bowel complications and provide appropriate treatments. Bowel complications can be caused by a variety of factors, including cancer, infection, and constipation.

Assessing for bowel complications:

- Observe the patient for signs of discomfort or distress, such as facial grimacing, moaning, or clutching their abdomen.

- Ask the patient about their bowel movements, including frequency, consistency, and presence of any blood or mucus.

- Palpate the abdomen to check for tenderness, swelling, or other abnormalities.

- Check the patient's vital signs, including heart rate, blood pressure, and body temperature, for any changes that may indicate a bowel complication.

- Monitor the patient's fluid and electrolyte levels, as imbalances can contribute to bowel complications.

- Ask the patient about their current medications, as some medications can cause constipation or other bowel complications.

Treating bowel complications:

- If the patient is constipated, try to increase their fluid and fiber intake to help regulate their bowel movements. This can include drinking plenty of water and eating high-fiber foods, such as fruits, vegetables, and whole grains.

- Administer laxatives or enemas as prescribed by the doctor to help relieve constipation.

- If the patient is experiencing diarrhea, focus on replacing lost fluids and electrolytes to prevent dehydration. This can include giving the patient clear fluids and electrolyte solutions, such as saline or Pedialyte.

- Administer antidiarrheal medications as prescribed by the doctor to help control diarrhea.

- If the patient has a bowel obstruction, surgical intervention may be necessary. The doctor will determine the appropriate treatment for this complication.

- Provide the patient with pain medication as needed to manage any discomfort associated with bowel complications.

Genitourinary Complications in the Hospice Patient

Genitourinary complications can be common in individuals with advanced illnesses or those who are immobile. One such complication is a urinary tract infection (UTI), which can be caused by bacteria entering the urinary system.

To assess for a UTI, the nurse will monitor the patient's urinary output, as well as look for any signs or symptoms of infection. This may include frequent or urgent urination, pain or burning during urination, cloudy or bloody urine, and discomfort in the lower abdominal or pelvic area.

If you suspect that a patient has a UTI, a urine sample must be obtained for testing to confirm the infection. This can be done through a clean catch urine sample, or in some cases, a catheter may be necessary to collect the sample.

Treatment for a UTI will depend on the severity of the infection and the overall health of the patient. In some cases, antibiotics may be prescribed to help clear the infection. The patient should be monitored closely for any changes in their symptoms and to adjust the treatment plan as necessary.

Managing a catheter can also be a part of preventing UTIs in patients who are unable to urinate on their own. This may be necessary for individuals who are bedridden or have mobility issues. To manage a catheter, keep the area clean and dry and monitor for any signs of infection or other complications.

Catheters are tubes that are inserted into the body for the purpose of draining fluids or administering medications. In hospice care, catheters may be used for a variety of purposes, including the management of incontinence, measurement of urine output, and relief of bladder distention.

There are several different types of catheters that may be used in hospice care, including:

- Intermittent catheters: These are catheters that are inserted into the bladder on a temporary basis to drain urine. They are typically used to manage incontinence or to measure urine output.

- Indwelling catheters: These are catheters that are left in place for an extended period of time, typically several days to a few weeks. They may be used to manage incontinence or to relieve bladder distention.

- Suprapubic catheters: These are catheters that are inserted through the abdomen into the bladder. They may be used as an alternative to urethral catheters in cases where urethral insertion is not possible or is not advisable.

- Condom catheters: These are catheters that are worn externally and are attached to a tube that drains urine into a bag. They may be used as an alternative to indwelling catheters in some cases.

The hospice nurse will carefully assess the need for a catheter and select the appropriate type based on the patient's individual needs and circumstances. The nurse should also be trained in proper insertion and care of the catheter, including infection prevention measures.

Infection control is an important consideration when managing urinary catheters in hospice care. *Catheter-associated urinary tract infections (CAUTIs)* are a common complication of catheterization and can cause serious morbidity and mortality in hospice patients.

To prevent CAUTIs and other infections, hospice nurse should follow recommended guidelines for infection control, including:

- Hand hygiene: Proper hand hygiene is essential for preventing the spread of infection. The nurse should wash their hands with soap and water or use an alcohol-based hand sanitizer before and after handling the catheter or other equipment.

- Sterile technique: When inserting or caring for the catheter, the nurse should use sterile technique to minimize the risk of infection. This may include the use of gloves, masks, and gowns.

- Catheter maintenance: The nurse should regularly check the catheter for signs of infection, such as redness or swelling at the insertion site, and should promptly report any concerns to the healthcare team. The nurse should also follow recommended guidelines for catheter care, including changing the catheter and collecting urine samples as needed.

- Patient education: The nurse should educate the patient and their family about the importance of infection control and the steps they can take to prevent infections, such as practicing good hygiene and not tampering with the catheter.

Proper infection control measures are essential for preventing CAUTIs and other infections in hospice patients with urinary catheters. The nurse should be diligent in following recommended guidelines and in educating the patient and their family about infection prevention.

In addition to catheterization, portable urinals may also be used in hospice care to manage incontinence and promote comfort. A *urinal* is a small, lightweight container that can be carried by the patient and used to collect urine when needed.

There are several different types of urinals that may be used in hospice care, including:

- Portable urinals: These are small, handheld containers that can be carried by the patient and used to collect urine when needed. They may be made of plastic or other materials and may have a lid to prevent spills.

- Bedside urinals: These are larger containers that are designed to be used at the patient's bedside. They may have a spout or other feature to facilitate easy drainage of urine.

- Female urinals: These are designed specifically for use by female patients and may be shaped differently to accommodate the female anatomy.

The use of urinals in hospice care can help to promote the patient's comfort and independence by allowing them to manage their own urinary needs without the need for assistance. It can also help to reduce the risk of infection and other complications associated with catheterization.

Case study: On the next visit, hospice case manager Sarah asked Mrs. Nesbitt if she had been drinking fluids. Mrs. Nesbitt and her daughter Janice reported that she had been very good about drinking a lot of water, but they were concerned because lately Mrs. Nesbitt's urine had been brown, and it was painful to go.

Sarah contacted Dr. Harris who ordered a urinalysis. Sarah retrieved a UA kit from her car-stock and obtained the sample from Mrs. Nesbitt. She then transported the sample to the lab, which reported Mrs. Nesbitt had blood in her urine and a confirmed urinary tract infection.

Dr. Harris called in a prescription to Mrs. Nesbitt's pharmacy and her daughter Janice picked it up and brought it to her mom. Sarah called Mrs. Nesbitt a few days later to check on her symptoms. She was relieved to hear that Mrs. Nesbitt no longer had any symptoms and was comfortably resting. Sarah thanked her for the update, and they made plans for Sarah to visit again the following Monday for a full visit.

Potential Respiratory Complications and Management

One common complication in hospice patients is respiratory distress, which can be caused by a variety of factors such as pneumonia, chronic obstructive pulmonary disease (COPD), or heart failure. Symptoms of respiratory distress include shortness of breath, rapid breathing, and an increased heart rate.

To manage respiratory distress, oxygen therapy may be used to improve the patient's oxygen levels. This can be administered using a nasal cannula or a face mask, depending on the severity of the patient's condition.

In addition to oxygen therapy, comfort kit medications such as opioids and benzodiazepines can be used to manage symptoms and improve the patient's overall comfort. These medications can help to reduce pain and anxiety and can also help to control symptoms such as cough and secretions.

The patient should be monitored for potential infections, as these can worsen their respiratory status and lead to further complications. Some common infections to watch for include pneumonia, influenza, and sepsis.

To identify these infections, the nurse should pay attention to the patient's vital signs and any changes in their symptoms. For example, a sudden worsening of shortness of breath or an increase in coughing could be a sign of pneumonia. Additionally, laboratory tests such as blood cultures and sputum cultures can be used to diagnose infections.

Once an infection is identified, it is critical to promptly initiate treatment. This can involve the use of antibiotics, and in some cases, hospitalization may be necessary. In addition to medical treatment, the nurse should also focus on providing supportive care to the patient, such as providing oxygen therapy and pain management.

Case study: Hospice nurse case manager Sarah knocked on Mrs. Nesbitt's door with no response. Sarah was concerned because she confirmed her appointment with Mrs. Nesbitt earlier in the day. She peered into the window and saw Mrs. Nesbitt sitting on the couch leaning forward with her elbows on her knees.

Mrs. Nesbitt saw Sarah and slowly shuffled to the door and opened it. She greeted Sarah but stated that she didn't know who Sarah was or why she was there.

Sarah noticed Mrs. Nesbitt's lips were blue and that she seemed out of breath. Sarah slowly and calmly reintroduced herself which effectively reoriented Mrs. Nesbitt.

Mrs. Nesbitt invited Sarah into her home, which Sarah noticed was disheveled and unkempt. Sarah made note of Mrs. Nesbitt's orientation and continued with her assessment. She checked Mrs. Nesbitt's oxygen saturation, which was below 90%.

Sarah checked Mrs. Nesbitt's medication orders and confirmed that Dr. Harris signed orders to use the oxygen concentrator the DME provider delivered upon admission, with 1-3 LPM as needed for shortness of breath. Mrs. Nesbitt consented to using oxygen with a nasal cannula, so Sarah administered the oxygen and continued to monitor Mrs. Nesbitt.

After several minutes of oxygen therapy, Mrs. Nesbitt reported she was beginning to feel better. Sarah asked her if she felt comfortable continuing her assessment, and she agreed to continue.

Mrs. Nesbitt admitted to using her rescue inhaler more frequently lately and reported that she felt more confused. She stated that her daughter had been ill and not able to visit for the last few days. Mrs. Nesbitt said she felt scared to call anyone, but she didn't remember the instructions for the oxygen concentrator.

Sarah provided Mrs. Nesbitt with emotional support and reassured her that she could call the phone number for the hospice provider 24 hours a day and a nurse would be able to help walk her through any difficulties or even make an after-hours visit if needed.

Mrs. Nesbitt felt much better and reported that she understood where to locate the number for the hospice provider. She agreed to call in the future and stated that it made her feel safer knowing that a nurse was available to her at any time she had an emergency.

Sarah provided Mrs. Nesbitt with written instructions for using the oxygen concentrator and went over Dr. Harris's orders for when to use it. Sarah also verified that signs were hung on the front door and in the house notifying visitors and reminding Mrs. Nesbitt that oxygen is in use and is highly flammable.

Sarah provided written oxygen safety instructions for Mrs. Nesbitt and had a discussion with her about everything she wrote down. Mrs. Nesbitt thanked Sarah for providing the instructions written and verbally as this was her preferred method of learning. Mrs. Nesbitt then said she heard Sarah say that she shouldn't use petroleum-based lip balm while using oxygen therapy and showed Sarah her lip balm. Sarah looked at the ingredient list and showed Mrs. Nesbitt that her lip balm was water-based, which made Mrs. Nesbitt happy that she could continue using it.

Sarah called Mrs. Nesbitt's daughter Janice and made a plan for Janice to call the hospice provider in the event she wouldn't be able to visit for extended periods. Sarah then called the hospice social worker Madilynn who agreed to visit Mrs. Nesbitt and assess her for any support she can offer. Sarah also called Dr. Harris to provide him with an update on Mrs. Nesbitt and to inform him that she had begun using oxygen therapy.

Cognitive Changes

The hospice nurse will regularly assess a patient's cognitive abilities and changes in their mental state as they near the end of life. This assessment can provide valuable information to the healthcare team and the patient's family, and it can help to ensure that the patient receives appropriate care and support.

One of the first signs of cognitive changes in a dying patient is a decrease in their level of consciousness. The patient may become drowsy or unresponsive, and they may no longer respond to stimuli such as voices or touch. In some cases, the patient may experience periods of delirium, with symptoms such as confusion, agitation, and hallucinations.

Another common sign of cognitive changes is a decline in the patient's ability to communicate. The patient may have difficulty speaking or understanding others, and they may become less communicative overall. They may also experience changes in their memory, with difficulty recalling recent events or information.

As the end of life approaches, the patient may also exhibit changes in their emotional state. They may become anxious or agitated, or they may experience feelings of fear or sadness. In some cases, the patient may express regret or remorse, or they may have difficulty accepting their impending death.

The hospice nurse will closely monitor the patient for these cognitive changes and will provide support and comfort as needed. The nurse should also communicate with the patient's family and other members of the care team about any changes in the patient's mental state and provide education and support to help them understand and cope with these changes.

In some cases, the hospice nurse may need to administer medications to control symptoms such as delirium or anxiety. The nurse should also work closely with the patient's healthcare provider to ensure that the patient's pain and other symptoms are managed effectively.

Musculoskeletal Changes

One of the common musculoskeletal changes in a dying patient is the development of contractures. *Contractures* are a condition in which the muscles and tendons become tight and shortened, leading to stiffness and difficulty moving the affected joints. This can cause discomfort and pain, and it can make it difficult for the patient to perform activities of daily living such as dressing, bathing, and eating.

Contractures can be caused by a variety of factors, including immobility, lack of exercise, and underlying medical conditions such as stroke or arthritis. They can also be a result of the natural processes of aging or the body's response to illness and stress.

To assess for contractures, the hospice nurse should carefully examine the patient's joints and muscles, looking for stiffness, decreased range of motion, and other signs of contractures. The nurse should also ask the patient about any pain or discomfort they are experiencing, and they should observe the patient during activities such as dressing and bathing.

Treatment for contractures may include medications to control pain and inflammation, physical therapy to stretch and loosen the affected muscles and tendons, and assistive devices such as splints or braces to support the joints and prevent further contractures. In some cases, the healthcare provider may recommend surgical intervention to release the contracted muscles and tendons.

To provide comfort and support to the patient with contractures, the hospice nurse should focus on maintaining the patient's mobility and independence. This may include providing assistive devices, helping the patient with exercises to stretch and loosen the affected muscles and tendons, and providing support and encouragement during activities of daily living. The nurse should also regularly assess and manage the patient's pain and other symptoms, and they should provide emotional support and comfort to the patient and their family.

Sociological Concerns

One of the common sociological concerns in a dying patient is the impact of the end of life on their family and loved ones. The patient's illness and impending death can be a source of stress, anxiety, and grief for their family, and it can affect their relationships, finances, and overall quality of life.

To assess for sociological concerns, the hospice nurse should carefully listen to the patient and their family, and they should ask open-ended questions to encourage them to talk about their feelings and concerns. The nurse should also observe the patient's family dynamic and interactions, looking for signs of stress, conflict, or other concerns.

Treatment for sociological concerns may involve providing support and resources to the patient's family, such as information on grief and bereavement, referrals to support groups and counseling services, and assistance with practical matters such as finances and end-of-life planning. In some cases, the healthcare provider may recommend interventions such as family therapy or mediation to address specific issues or conflicts within the family.

Case study: Case manager Sarah received a call from Janice, Mrs. Nesbitt's daughter. Janice was crying and upset because she had gotten into a fight with her sister Tammy who recently learned that her mother had signed a Do Not Resuscitate order when she was admitted to hospice. Janice expressed her concerns about her sister Tammy's understanding and acceptance of her mother's DNR.

Sarah, understanding the gravity of the situation, offered to meet Janice and Tammy at Mrs. Nesbitt's house to help explain the situation and provide support. She also suggested involving the hospice's social worker, Madilynn, in the meeting as she believed Madilynn's expertise in the field would be beneficial in helping Tammy understand and come to terms with the DNR. Janice agreed to Sarah's suggestion and Madilynn agreed to meet Sarah at Mrs. Nesbitt's house.

Sarah and Madilynn arrived at Mrs. Nesbitt's house and met with Janice and Tammy. They explained the purpose and implications of a DNR, which is a legal document that states their mother's wishes not to receive cardiopulmonary resuscitation (CPR) or other life-sustaining treatments in the event her heart stops, or she stops breathing. They also emphasized that the DNR is in place to honor their mother's autonomy and respect her wishes and that it is not a decision made lightly.

Sarah and Madilynn also provided emotional support and guidance to both Janice and Tammy, addressing their concerns and answering any questions they had. They also provided information on the other palliative care options available to help alleviate symptoms and improve their mom's quality of life.

In the end, Tammy was able to understand and accept her mother's DNR and was able to focus on being present and spending quality time with her mom. Sarah and Madilynn continued to provide support and monitor the situation, ensuring that the family had the information and support they needed during this difficult time.

Throughout the process, Sarah and Madilynn were respectful of the patient's autonomy, while also providing emotional support to the family. They were able to provide clear information on the DNR and other palliative care options, addressing the concerns and questions of the family members. They also helped the family understand the importance of honoring their mom's wishes and respecting her autonomy. This ultimately led to a more peaceful and comfortable end-of-life experience for both Mrs. Nesbitt and her daughters.

Assess Spiritual Needs

To assess for spiritual needs, the hospice nurse should carefully listen to the patient and their family, and they should ask open-ended questions to encourage them to talk about their beliefs, values, and spiritual concerns. The nurse should also observe the patient's behavior and interactions, looking for signs of spiritual distress or discomfort.

A patient with spiritual concerns may require support and resources, such as referrals to chaplains or other spiritual care providers, assistance with prayer or meditation, and support for the patient's religious or spiritual practices. In some cases, the healthcare provider may recommend interventions such as spiritual counseling or support groups to address specific spiritual needs or concerns.

It is important for the hospice nurse to communicate openly and honestly with the patient and their family about their spiritual needs and to provide empathy and support. The nurse should also work closely with the chaplain and other members of the healthcare team to coordinate care and ensure that the patient's spiritual needs are met.

Case study: As her health continued to decline, Mrs. Nesbitt began to express concerns about her soul after death. She shared with Sarah that she was agnostic and had never been particularly religious, but she was still struggling with the idea of what would happen to her after she passed away. Sarah listened attentively and reassured Mrs. Nesbitt that her feelings were normal and that there were resources available to help her find peace and acceptance in the end-of-life process.

To address Mrs. Nesbitt's concerns, Sarah reached out to the hospice chaplain, Jacob, who met Sarah at Mrs. Nesbitt's house. Jacob was a non-denominational chaplain who provided spiritual guidance to patients of all beliefs.

During the meeting, Jacob listened to Mrs. Nesbitt's concerns and provided her with a non-denominational perspective on death and the afterlife. He explained that the end of life is a journey and that there is no one right or wrong way to approach it. He also assured her that there is no need to have all the answers, but rather the importance is to have a sense of peace and acceptance about her life coming to an end.

Jacob also provided Mrs. Nesbitt with resources such as literature and music that she could use to reflect on her life and her impending death. He also gave her an opportunity to ask any questions she might have, and to express any fears or concerns she had about death.

As the meeting came to a close, Mrs. Nesbitt felt a sense of peace and acceptance about her life coming to an end. She expressed her gratitude to Jacob and Sarah for their support and guidance. She felt reassured that she was not alone in her thoughts and feelings and that there were resources available to help her find peace and acceptance in the end-of-life process. She was able to spend her remaining days with a sense of serenity, surrounded by the love and support of her family and the hospice team.

Assess the Patient's Ability to Perform Activities of Daily Living (ADLs)

To assess a patient's ability to perform ADLs, the hospice nurse should carefully observe the patient and ask them about their daily routine and activities. The nurse should look for signs of difficulty with self-care tasks such as bathing, dressing, and eating, as well as more complex activities such as managing medications, cooking, and performing household chores.

The hospice nurse will evaluate the need to provide support and assistance from a Home Health Aide or CNA. In some cases, the healthcare provider may recommend additional interventions or equipment, such as assistive devices or modifications to the patient's home, to help the patient perform ADLs more easily. The nurse should also provide education and support to the patient and their family on how to manage the patient's care and maintain their safety and comfort. It is important for the hospice nurse to communicate openly and honestly with the patient and their family about their ability to perform ADLs and to provide support and guidance.

Case study: As Sarah continued to visit Mrs. Nesbitt, she noticed that her appearance had changed. During her last three visits, Mrs. Nesbitt had worn the same clothes and her hair seemed greasy and her skin looked dirty. Sarah was concerned and asked Mrs. Nesbitt if she had been able to bathe regularly. Mrs. Nesbitt admitted that she had been having difficulty with that and other activities of daily living (ADLs) due to her declining health.

Sarah knew that maintaining personal hygiene and grooming is an important aspect of comfort and well-being for patients nearing the end of their lives. She quickly identified that Mrs. Nesbitt needed assistance with her ADLs and discussed this with her and her family. They agreed that it would be beneficial for her to receive help with her ADLs.

Sarah then arranged for the home health aide Jennifer to visit with Mrs. Nesbitt every Monday, Wednesday, and Friday to help her with her bathing and other ADLs needs. Jennifer arrived promptly and assisted Mrs. Nesbitt with her showering, grooming, getting dressed and other personal care needs. She also helped with other tasks such as preparing meals, light housekeeping, and laundry. This support allowed Mrs. Nesbitt to maintain her independence and dignity while receiving the necessary assistance.

Sarah also discussed with Mrs. Nesbitt other interventions that can improve comfort, such as positioning, skin care, and oral hygiene. She also provided education on how to prevent bedsores and pressure ulcers, as well as how to prevent and manage other symptoms such as pain, constipation, and fatigue.

Sarah also made sure to communicate with the rest of the hospice team, including the physician, nurse, and social worker, about the changes in Mrs. Nesbitt's condition and needs, and to ensure a coordinated and comprehensive care plan.

With the help of the home health aide, Mrs. Nesbitt was able to maintain her personal hygiene and grooming, which improved her comfort and overall well-being. She felt more confident, and her family noticed a positive change in her mood and appearance. Sarah and the hospice team continued to monitor her condition and adjust the care plan as needed to meet her changing needs.

Additionally, Sarah also made sure that Mrs. Nesbitt's family was educated and supported in their role as caregivers, providing them with resources and guidance on how to assist her with her ADLs and other needs, and helping them to understand the importance of maintaining personal hygiene and grooming for their loved one's comfort and well-being during the end-of-life journey.

As Jennifer continued to assist Mrs. Nesbitt with her ADLs and other needs, an unexpected side benefit emerged. Over time, Jennifer and Mrs. Nesbitt grew closer. Their interactions were not limited to just providing care, but also included conversations and spending time together.

Jennifer was able to provide emotional support and companionship, which was important for Mrs. Nesbitt who was facing the end of her life. Mrs. Nesbitt appreciated Jennifer's kind and compassionate nature and found comfort in her company. They talked about their shared interests and reminisced about their past experiences. Jennifer also provided her with emotional support and listened to her concerns and fears, which helped Mrs. Nesbitt feel less alone during this difficult time.

Mrs. Nesbitt also enjoyed having someone to share her day-to-day life with and this companionship helped to improve her mood and overall well-being. As a result, Jennifer's presence brought a positive change to Mrs. Nesbitt and her family, providing her with a sense of comfort and companionship during the end-of-life journey.

Sarah noticed the positive impact of their relationship and provided guidance and support for Jennifer to ensure that the relationship between the two of them was safe, healthy, and beneficial for both. And this relationship between Jennifer and Mrs. Nesbitt was not only beneficial for Mrs. Nesbitt but also for Jennifer, as it allowed her to form a connection and bond with a patient in a way that is not always possible, and it also helped to make her work as a home health aide more meaningful and fulfilling.

Durable Medical Equipment (DME)

Durable Medical Equipment (DME) is an essential component of hospice care. It includes a wide range of equipment and supplies that are used to provide comfort, support, and independence to patients nearing the end of their lives. The use of DME can be critical in managing symptoms and improving the patient's quality of life.

One of the most common types of DME provided in hospice care is the hospital bed. Hospice patients often require a hospital bed to provide a higher level of comfort and support than a traditional bed. Hospital beds are adjustable, allowing patients to be positioned in a variety of ways to prevent bedsores and promote comfort. They also typically have a built-in mattress that can be adjusted for firmness, as well as side rails to provide safety and support.

Another common type of DME provided in hospice care is oxygen equipment. Patients with chronic respiratory diseases such as COPD may require oxygen therapy to help them breathe more easily and to manage their symptoms. Oxygen therapy can be provided through a variety of devices such as nasal cannulas, face masks, or non-invasive ventilators. The type of oxygen equipment used will depend on the patient's specific needs and the severity of their condition.

Patients with mobility issues may require assistive devices such as wheelchairs, walkers, or canes. These devices can help patients to maintain their independence and mobility, as well as provide them with the support they need to safely move around their home. In addition, patients who are bedbound may require lift equipment and slings to aid with transfers, repositioning, and activities of daily living.

Another important type of DME that is commonly provided in hospice care is incontinence supplies. Patients nearing the end of their lives may require assistance with managing their incontinence. Incontinence supplies such as adult briefs (we don't say diapers), pads, and underpads (chux) can be provided to help patients maintain their dignity and comfort.

Finally, hospice patients may also require other types of DME such as suction machines, nebulizers, and feeding pumps, depending on their specific needs. Suction machines can be used to remove secretions from the airways of patients with respiratory issues, nebulizers can be used to administer medication to patients with respiratory issues and feeding pumps can be used to provide nutrition to patients who are unable to eat or swallow.

It's worth noting that DME providers are different from hospice providers, so when a hospice patient requires DME, the patient's hospice care team will work with a DME supplier to provide the necessary equipment, and the DME supplier will handle the logistics of delivering, setting up, and maintaining the equipment.

To assess for a patient's DME needs, the hospice nurse should carefully evaluate the patient's physical condition and functional abilities. The nurse should consider the patient's medical diagnosis, current symptoms, and potential future needs, and they should ask the patient and their family about any equipment or assistive devices that the patient is currently using or may require in the future.

The nurse will coordinate care with the DME supplier to provide the necessary equipment and assistive devices. The nurse should work closely with the DME supplier to ensure that the patient receives the appropriate equipment in a timely manner and that it is properly fitted and adjusted to meet their needs.

In some cases, the healthcare provider may recommend additional interventions or equipment, such as oxygen therapy or mobility aids, to help the patient maintain their independence and quality of life. The nurse should provide education and support to the patient and their family on how to use the equipment safely and effectively.

In summary, DME plays an important role in hospice care by providing comfort, support, and independence to patients nearing the end of their lives. Common types of DME include hospital beds, oxygen equipment, assistive devices, incontinence supplies, suction machines, nebulizers, and feeding pumps. The specific DME provided to a patient will depend on their individual needs and the severity of their condition. It is important for the hospice care team to work with DME suppliers to ensure that patients receive the appropriate equipment and support they need to manage their symptoms and improve their quality of life.

Pain Assessment and Symptom Management with the Comfort Kit

Pain control is an important aspect of care for the dying patient. When left unmanaged, pain can significantly impact the patient's quality of life, causing them to experience physical and emotional suffering. Therefore, it is important to proactively address pain in the dying patient and stay in front of it to ensure that it is adequately managed.

One way to proactively manage pain in the dying patient is to use a pain scale to regularly assess the patient's pain levels. This can help the healthcare team determine the most appropriate interventions to control the pain. It is also important to involve the patient and their loved ones in the pain management process, as they can provide valuable insight into the patient's pain experience and preferences for treatment.

Hospice nurses use a variety of pain scales to assess the level of pain experienced by a dying patient. Some common types of pain scales include:

- Numeric Rating Scale (NRS): This scale asks the patient to rate their pain on a scale from 0 to 10, with 0 being no pain and 10 being the worst pain imaginable.

- Verbal Rating Scale (VRS): This scale asks the patient to describe their pain using words, such as mild, moderate, or severe.

- Visual Analog Scale (VAS): This scale consists of a line with two anchor points, one representing no pain and the other representing the worst pain imaginable. The patient is asked to mark their pain level on the line.

- Faces Pain Scale (FPS): This scale consists of a series of faces that range from happy (no pain) to sad (worst pain imaginable). The patient is asked to choose the face that best represents their pain level.

- Wong-Baker FACES Pain Rating Scale: This scale is similar to the FPS but includes a series of faces with different expressions, ranging from a happy face (no pain) to a crying face (worst pain imaginable). The patient is asked to choose the face that best represents their pain level.

Hospice nurses may use one or more of these scales when assessing the dying patient for pain. The scale chosen may depend on the patient's age, cognitive abilities, and communication abilities. It is important to regularly assess the patient's pain level and response to treatment to ensure that the pain is being effectively managed.

It is important to individualize the approach to pain management in the dying patient and consider the patient's preferences and needs. The healthcare team should work with the patient and their loved ones to determine the most appropriate methods for pain control. It is also important to regularly assess the patient's pain levels and response to treatment to ensure that the pain is being effectively managed. By staying in front of the pain proactively, the healthcare team can help the dying patient maintain a sense of comfort and dignity during this difficult time.

Pharmacologic methods of pain relief include the use of medications, such as nonsteroidal anti-inflammatory drugs (NSAIDs), opioids, and acetaminophen. It is important for hospice case managers to work with the patient's healthcare team to determine the most appropriate medication and dosage, as well as to monitor for any potential side effects.

The hospice comfort kit is a set of medications that are commonly used in hospice care to manage symptoms and improve the patient's quality of life. These medications are typically provided by the hospice agency and are intended for use in the patient's home. The hospice comfort kit typically includes a variety of medications that can be used to manage pain, shortness of breath, constipation, nausea, and other common symptoms.

One of the most common medications in the hospice comfort kit is *morphine*, which is a strong opioid pain medication. Morphine is a powerful opioid pain medication that is often used in hospice care to manage moderate to severe pain and respiratory distress. It is typically administered orally.

Morphine works by binding to opioid receptors in the brain and spinal cord, which helps to block pain signals and increase the release of pain-reducing chemicals, such as endorphins. It is an effective pain medication for many types of pain, including cancer-related pain and pain from other terminal illnesses.

In addition to managing pain, morphine can also be used to manage respiratory distress in the dying patient. It can help to relax the muscles of the airways and improve breathing, which can provide significant comfort for the patient.

While morphine can be very effective in relieving pain, it can also cause side effects, including constipation, nausea, and drowsiness. It is important for the hospice case manager to monitor the patient for these side effects and work with the healthcare team to manage them as needed.

Morphine is contraindicated in patients with a history of hypersensitivity to morphine or other opioids, as well as in patients with severe respiratory depression or uncontrolled asthma. It should also be used with caution in patients with a history of drug abuse or addiction.

Liquid morphine is the most often used form of morphine in hospice care to manage pain and other symptoms in the dying patient. It is usually administered buccal or sublingual and can be a highly effective means of providing rapid symptom relief in the terminal phase of illness.

However, it is important for the hospice nurse to carefully assess the need for liquid morphine and to closely monitor the patient for any adverse effects or complications.

One of the most serious risks associated with liquid morphine is respiratory depression, which can occur when the medication slows down breathing. The nurse should monitor the patient's respiratory status closely and take steps to prevent or manage respiratory depression as needed.

Overall, the use of morphine can be an important aspect of hospice care and can provide significant symptom relief for the dying patient. However, it is important for the nurse to carefully assess the need for the medication, monitor the patient for any adverse effects or complications, and take appropriate steps to manage these risks.

Another common medication in the hospice comfort kit is *lorazepam*, which is a benzodiazepine used to manage anxiety and agitation. Lorazepam is typically given by mouth and may be used to help the patient relax and sleep. It is commonly used in hospice care to manage symptoms such as anxiety, agitation, and insomnia.

Lorazepam works by enhancing the effects of a neurotransmitter called GABA, which helps to calm the nervous system and reduce anxiety. It is typically taken orally but can also be given topically, intravenously, or rectally.

While lorazepam can be effective in managing symptoms, it can also cause side effects, such as drowsiness, dizziness, and impaired coordination. It is important for the hospice case manager to monitor the patient for these side effects and work with the healthcare team to manage them as needed.

Lorazepam is contraindicated in patients with a history of hypersensitivity to benzodiazepines or a history of narrow-angle glaucoma. It should also be used with caution in patients with a history of drug abuse or addiction.

Hyoscyamine is a medication that is commonly used in hospice care to manage symptoms such as excess oral secretions and discomfort related to gastrointestinal conditions. Excess oral secretions, also known as sialorrhea or drooling, can be a common symptom in hospice patients and can be caused by a variety of factors, including medications, neurological conditions, or difficulty swallowing. Hyoscyamine works by reducing the production of saliva and other fluids in the mouth and throat, which can help to alleviate discomfort and improve the quality of life for patients.

Excess oral secretions are sometimes called *"death rattles"* due to their production of a rattle-like sound due to secretions accumulating in the throat. This can be distressing for both the patient and their family.

The death rattle is a result of the muscles in the throat and chest relaxing as the patient approaches the end of life. This relaxation can cause secretions to accumulate in the throat, leading to the production of the rattle-like sound. In some cases, the death rattle may be accompanied by other symptoms, such as difficulty swallowing, coughing, or shortness of breath.

It is important to note that each patient's experience with the death rattle may be different. Some patients may be more aware of their surroundings and more able to communicate their needs, while others may be less responsive. In either case, the healthcare team should work to provide the best possible care and support to the patient and their family.

The case manager will perform a thorough assessment of the patient prior to administration, as hyoscyamine can have potential side effects and contraindications. For example, hyoscyamine can cause drowsiness and may interact with other medications, so it is important to carefully review the patient's medication list before prescribing it. In addition, hyoscyamine is not recommended for use in patients with certain conditions, such as narrow-angle glaucoma, severe ulcerative colitis, or a history of allergic reactions to atropine or similar medications.

If hyoscyamine is not appropriate or effective for a particular patient, there are several alternative medications that may be considered. These may include other anticholinergic medications, such as glycopyrrolate or scopolamine, or medications that target specific symptoms, such as nausea or vomiting. The hospice care team should work closely with the patient and their family to determine the most appropriate treatment approach based on the patient's individual needs and preferences.

Ondansetron is a medication commonly used in hospice care to manage nausea and vomiting. It is a type of antiemetic, which means it helps to prevent or reduce nausea and vomiting caused by chemotherapy, radiation therapy, or surgery. Ondansetron works by blocking the action of a chemical in the body called serotonin, which is involved in the control of nausea and vomiting.

Ondansetron is typically given as a tablet or oral solution, although it can also be given as an injection or suppository. It is generally well-tolerated, with common side effects including constipation, headache, and dizziness.

In hospice care, ondansetron may be used to manage nausea and vomiting caused by a variety of factors, including advanced cancer, kidney failure, and liver disease. It may also be used to manage nausea and vomiting associated with medications, such as opioids, which are commonly used in hospice care to manage pain.

Ondansetron is generally considered a safe and effective medication for managing nausea and vomiting in hospice care. However, it is important to carefully follow the dosing instructions provided by the hospice care team and to report any side effects to the healthcare provider. In some cases, alternative medications may be necessary to manage nausea and vomiting in hospice patients. These alternatives may include other antiemetics, such as promethazine or prochlorperazine, or medications to manage underlying conditions, such as acid-reducing agents for nausea caused by acid reflux.

Acetaminophen is a common pain reliever that is often used in hospice care to manage pain and discomfort, as well as elevated body temperature or fever. It is typically given orally, but in some cases, a suppository form may be used.
A *suppository* is a medication that is inserted into the rectum or vagina, where it is absorbed into the bloodstream. The use of a suppository may be preferred in hospice patients who are unable to swallow or who are experiencing nausea or vomiting, as it allows the medication to be absorbed directly into the bloodstream without the need for oral ingestion.

Acetaminophen suppositories are typically used to manage mild to moderate pain and may be used in conjunction with other pain medications. They are contraindicated in patients with liver disease or those who are allergic to acetaminophen.

Hospice caregivers must follow the dosing instructions provided by the patient's healthcare provider when administering acetaminophen suppositories. Overdosing on acetaminophen can be dangerous and can lead to liver damage which can be very painful and fatal. It is also important to note that acetaminophen is a non-opioid pain medication and should not be used as a replacement for opioid pain medication in patients who are already taking opioids for pain management.

Acetaminophen may be used when the patient is experiencing discomfort from terminal fever. *Terminal fever*, also known as the "terminal phase fever," is a phenomenon that can occur in patients who are dying or near the end of life. It is characterized by a sudden, unexplained increase in body temperature, often to levels that are higher than what is considered normal. Terminal fever is not a specific illness or condition, but rather a symptom that can occur as the body's natural functions begin to shut down.

It is important to note that each patient's experience with terminal fever may be different. Some patients may experience fever for a short period of time, while others may have ongoing fever for several days or weeks. In either case, the healthcare team should work to provide the best possible care and support to the patient and their family.

Bisacodyl suppository is a medication that is used to stimulate bowel movements in patients with constipation. It is typically used in hospice care to help manage symptoms of constipation that can be common in patients with terminal illnesses. Bisacodyl suppository works by increasing the contraction of the muscles in the intestine, which helps to move stool through the bowel more effectively.

It is important for the hospice nurse to carefully consider the use of bisacodyl suppository, as it can cause side effects such as abdominal cramping and bloating. It should not be used in patients with certain medical conditions, such as severe abdominal pain or inflammatory bowel disease. The nurse should also be aware of any potential interactions with other medications the patient may be taking.

If the patient is experiencing constipation, the hospice nurse may try other methods of relieving symptoms before resorting to a bisacodyl suppository. These methods may include increasing fluid intake, encouraging the patient to be physically active, and adding fiber to the patient's diet. If these methods are not effective, the nurse may consider using a different medication or combination of medications to manage the patient's constipation.

Oxygen therapy is often used in hospice care to help manage symptoms such as shortness of breath and fatigue. It is typically administered through a nasal cannula or a face mask and can be delivered continuously or on an as-needed basis.

There are several considerations to take into account when using oxygen in hospice care. The first is the patient's oxygen saturation level, which can be measured using a pulse oximeter. If the patient's oxygen saturation level is below a certain threshold, oxygen therapy may be recommended to help improve their oxygenation.

Another consideration is the patient's ability to tolerate oxygen therapy. Some patients may experience discomfort or irritation when using oxygen and may need to adjust the flow rate or switch to a different delivery method to find relief. It is important to monitor the patient's response to oxygen therapy and make any necessary adjustments.

Contraindications to oxygen therapy in hospice care include certain medical conditions, such as carbon monoxide poisoning or an overactive thyroid gland. It is important to review the patient's medical history and consider any potential contraindications before starting oxygen therapy.

Oxygen safety is an important aspect of healthcare, particularly in hospice settings where patients may be using oxygen therapy. It is essential for caregivers and facilities to be properly educated on oxygen safety measures in order to prevent accidents and ensure the well-being of patients. A hospice case manager can play a key role in providing this education, which may include topics such as proper handling and storage of oxygen tanks, the proper use of oxygen masks and nasal cannulas, and the importance of keeping the oxygen source away from sources of ignition such as cigarettes or open flames.

Patients and caregivers should be educated on the use of water-based lubricants and lotions and avoiding other common flammable household items, particularly petroleum-based products. It is also important to have protocols in place for responding to oxygen emergencies, such as leaks or fires. By providing education and training on oxygen safety, hospice case managers can help to ensure the safe and effective use of oxygen therapy for patients in their care.

In hospice care, the use of morphine, lorazepam, and other comfort medications should be guided by the patient's goals of care and preferences. The hospice case manager should work with the patient and their family to determine the appropriate dose and frequency of comfort medications and should adjust the medication as needed to ensure that the patient's symptoms are well-controlled. The case manager should also communicate with the patient and their family about the potential benefits and risks of using these medications and should involve them in decision-making about their use.

In addition to medication, non-pharmacologic methods can be used to manage pain in the dying patient. These methods may include relaxation techniques, such as deep breathing and visualization; therapeutic touch; acupuncture; heat and cold therapy; and music therapy. These methods can be used alone or in combination with medication to provide relief.

Case study: During Sarah's next visit to Mrs. Nesbitt's home, she noticed a significant change in her condition. Mrs. Nesbitt was experiencing increased respiratory distress and was having difficulty breathing. Janice, who was staying with her mother now, expressed her concerns and fears about her mother's worsening condition.

Sarah assessed Mrs. Nesbitt's condition and found that her oxygen saturation levels were low, and her respiratory rate was elevated. She discussed the situation with the hospice physician, and they agreed that it was time to provide Mrs. Nesbitt with a comfort kit of medications.

Sarah provided education to Janice on how to use the comfort kit medications, including the indications for use as well as contraindications. She also provided specific instructions on how to manage Mrs. Nesbitt's symptoms using the comfort kit medications.

Sarah instructed Janice to administer medication such as morphine sulfate to help manage her mother's pain and to reduce her respiratory distress. Morphine is a strong opioid pain medication that works by changing the way the brain and nervous system respond to pain. It is typically administered in hospice in concentrate form via the sublingual or buccal route. It is important to note that Morphine should be used with caution in patients with respiratory conditions as it can suppress breathing. Sarah provided instructions on how to monitor Mrs. Nesbitt's breathing rate and oxygen saturation levels and to adjust the dosage as needed.

She also provided instructions on how to administer medication such as lorazepam, which can help to reduce anxiety and agitation. Lorazepam is a benzodiazepine medication that works by increasing the activity of a chemical called GABA in the brain. It is typically administered by oral or intravenous routes. It is important to note that Lorazepam can cause drowsiness and sedation, so it is important to monitor the patient's level of consciousness and adjust the dosage as needed.

Sarah also provided guidance on how to administer hyoscyamine, which can be used to help reduce excess oral secretions. Hyoscyamine is an anticholinergic medication that works by blocking the action of a chemical called acetylcholine in the body. It is typically administered by oral or sublingual routes. It is important to note that Hyoscyamine can cause dry mouth, constipation, and blurred vision, so it is important to monitor the patient for these side effects and adjust the dosage as needed.

Sarah also provided guidance on how to administer ondansetron which can be used to prevent or treat nausea and vomiting. Ondansetron is a serotonin 5-HT3 receptor antagonist medication that works by blocking the action of serotonin, a chemical messenger in the body that can cause nausea and vomiting. It is typically administered by oral or rectal routes. It is important to note that Ondansetron can cause constipation, headache, and dizziness so it is important to monitor the patient for these side effects and adjust the dosage as needed.

Sarah provided guidance on how to administer acetaminophen to help manage pain. Acetaminophen is a medication that works by blocking the production of certain chemicals in the body that cause pain and inflammation. It is typically administered by oral or rectal routes. It is important to note that Acetaminophen can cause liver damage if taken in large doses or if used for long periods of time, so it is important to monitor the patient's liver function and adjust the dosage as needed.

Sarah discussed the importance of monitoring Mrs. Nesbitt's vital signs, including her oxygen saturation levels and respiratory rate, and instructed Janice on when to administer the medication based on these vital signs. She also provided guidance on how to adjust the dosage of the medications based on the patient's response.

Sarah also informed Janice that the hospice team is available 24/7 to provide support and guidance and encouraged her to reach out to them if she had any questions or concerns. Sarah provided detailed documentation of the visit and the care provided to Mrs. Nesbitt and made sure that all the team members were updated on her condition and the interventions made.

With the guidance provided by Sarah, Janice felt more confident in managing her mother's symptoms and providing her with the comfort and support she needed during this difficult time. Mrs. Nesbitt's comfort and quality of life improved with the use of the comfort kit medications and her family was able to feel more at ease knowing that they were providing the best possible care for their loved one. With the use of the comfort kit medications, Mrs. Nesbitt was able to experience a greater sense of peace and comfort as her symptoms were better managed.

It's important to note that the use of comfort kit medications is not intended to prolong the patient's life, but rather to alleviate symptoms and improve the patient's quality of life. The hospice team closely monitors the patient's condition and adjusts the medications as needed to ensure that the patient remains comfortable.

Non-Pharmacologic Pain Relief

Non-pharmacologic pain control refers to methods of managing pain that do not involve the use of medications. These methods can be particularly useful in the care of a dying patient, as they can provide relief without the potential for negative side effects or interactions with other medications the patient may be taking.

Relaxation techniques are a non-pharmacologic method of pain control that can be effective in reducing pain and improving the patient's overall sense of well-being. These techniques work by reducing muscle tension, calming the mind, and promoting a sense of relaxation.

Deep breathing is a simple relaxation technique that can be performed by the patient at any time. To perform deep breathing, the patient should be encouraged to find a comfortable position, either lying down or seated and focus on taking slow, deep breaths. The patient should inhale through their nose, hold their breath for a moment, and exhale slowly through their mouth. Deep breathing can help to slow the heart rate and lower blood pressure, which can in turn help to reduce pain.

Progressive muscle relaxation is another relaxation technique that involves tensing and relaxing specific muscle groups in the body. To perform this technique, the patient can be guided through tensing and relaxing each muscle group, starting with the feet and working up to the head. This technique can help to reduce muscle tension and promote relaxation.

Visualization is a relaxation technique that involves closing the eyes and imagining a peaceful scene or situation. The patient can be encouraged to visualize a place or situation that brings them a sense of calm and tranquility. Visualization can help to distract the patient from their pain and promote relaxation.

Therapeutic touch, also known as healing touch, is a non-pharmacologic method of pain control that involves the practitioner using their hands to transmit a sense of calm and well-being to the patient. This method is based on the belief that the practitioner can use their hands to manipulate the patient's energy field and promote healing.

To perform therapeutic touch, the practitioner typically stands near the patient and places their hands on or near the patient's body in a gentle, comforting manner. The practitioner may use a light touch or a gentle massage to transmit a sense of calm and relaxation to the patient. The goal of therapeutic touch is to promote relaxation and reduce stress, which may in turn help to reduce pain.

Therapeutic touch can be performed by trained practitioners, such as nurses, physical therapists, and massage therapists. It is typically used in conjunction with other forms of treatment, such as medication, to provide pain relief.

Music therapy is a non-pharmacologic method of pain control that involves using music to manage pain and improve the patient's overall sense of well-being. Music has been shown to have a number of benefits for pain management, including reducing anxiety, promoting relaxation, and providing a sense of distraction from the pain.

To perform music therapy, the patient can be provided with headphones and asked to listen to their favorite music, or a selection of calming tunes chosen by the patient or a loved one. It is important to consider the patient's preferences and needs when selecting music for therapy. Some patients may find classical music or nature sounds to be particularly calming, while others may prefer more upbeat or energetic music.

Music therapy can be performed by a trained music therapist or by the patient themselves with the guidance of a healthcare professional. It can be used alone or in combination with other forms of treatment, such as medication, to provide pain relief.

Non-pharmacologic pain control methods should typically be used in conjunction with, rather than as a replacement for, pharmacologic methods as prescribed by a healthcare provider. By using a combination of both pharmacologic and non-pharmacologic methods, it may be possible to achieve more effective pain management for the dying patient.

It is important to communicate with the patient and their healthcare team to determine the best approach for managing their pain. It may take some trial and error to find the right combination of methods that work best for the patient. It is important to individualize the approach to pain management in the dying patient and consider the patient's preferences and needs. The healthcare team should work with the patient and their loved ones to determine the most appropriate methods for pain control. It is also important to regularly assess the patient's pain levels and response to treatment to ensure that the pain is being effectively managed.

Case study: During Sarah's visit, Janice and her sister Tammy requested information on non-pharmacologic symptom control for Mrs. Nesbitt. They were interested in alternative methods to manage her symptoms and improve her comfort. Sarah discussed several specific non-pharmacologic methods of symptom relief for Mrs. Nesbitt's COPD and CHF with Janice and Tammy during her next visit.

First, she discussed the importance of pulmonary rehabilitation. This program includes exercises to improve lung function and muscle strength, as well as education on managing COPD symptoms such as breathing techniques and energy conservation strategies. Sarah provided instruction on specific exercises that Mrs. Nesbitt could do at home and encouraged Janice and Tammy to assist her in implementing a daily routine.

Next, Sarah discussed the use of oxygen therapy for Mrs. Nesbitt's COPD. She explained that providing oxygen can help to alleviate shortness of breath and improve her overall quality of life. Sarah provided instruction on how to properly set up and use the oxygen equipment and emphasized the importance of monitoring oxygen levels and adjusting the flow rate as needed.

Sarah also discussed the importance of regular chest physical therapy to help clear mucus from the lungs and improve breathing for Mrs. Nesbitt. She provided instruction on how to do specific chest physical therapy techniques such as deep breathing exercises, postural drainage, and vibration.

For CHF, Sarah discussed the importance of fluid management and lifestyle modifications such as reducing salt intake and weight management. Sarah provided instruction on how to monitor fluid intake and output, and how to recognize signs of fluid overload such as shortness of breath, swelling and weight gain.

Finally, Sarah discussed the importance of good sleep hygiene for Mrs. Nesbitt. She provided instruction on how to create a comfortable and relaxing sleep environment, such as maintaining a comfortable temperature in the room, minimizing noise, and using soft lighting. She also discussed the benefits of relaxation techniques such as progressive muscle relaxation and deep breathing exercises to promote a peaceful night's sleep.

Sarah emphasized the importance of monitoring Mrs. Nesbitt's condition, adjusting the interventions as needed, and the availability of the hospice team for support and guidance, encouraging Janice and Tammy to reach out to them if they had any questions or concerns.

Trajectories of the Dying Patient

The term "trajectory" is often used to refer to the course of a patient's illness or the general direction in which their health is headed. In the context of a dying patient, the trajectory of their illness can refer to the overall pattern of their condition, including any ups and downs and the rate at which their health is deteriorating.

Understanding a patient's trajectory can be helpful for the hospice team in predicting how the patient's condition is likely to progress and in planning for their care and support. It can also be helpful for the patient and their family in understanding what to expect and in making decisions about the patient's care and treatment.

There are several different trajectories that a dying patient may follow, including a rapid decline, a slow decline, periods of stability, unexpected complications, and sudden death. It is important for the hospice team to be aware of these different trajectories and to work with the patient and their family to provide the best possible care and support throughout the dying process.

Some patients may experience a swift decline in their condition, with their health deteriorating rapidly over a short period of time. Rapid decline refers to a quick deterioration in a patient's health, often over a period of days or weeks. This may be due to factors such as the progression of a terminal illness or complications related to treatment. This can be a distressing time for both the patient and their loved ones, as it can be difficult to cope with the sudden changes in the patient's condition.

There are many factors that can contribute to rapid decline in a patient's health. Some common illnesses that can cause rapid decline include:

- Cancer: Advanced cancer can cause rapid decline in a patient's health as the cancer spreads and becomes more difficult to treat.

- Sepsis: Sepsis is a severe and potentially life-threatening complication of an infection. It can cause rapid decline in a patient's condition as the body's immune system begins to attack healthy tissue and organs.

- Acute respiratory distress syndrome (ARDS): ARDS is a severe lung condition that can occur as a result of an infection, injury, or other medical condition. It can cause rapid decline in a patient's condition as the lungs become inflamed and filled with fluid, making it difficult to breathe.

- Organ failure: Rapid decline can also occur when a patient's organs begin to fail, such as the heart, kidneys, or liver. This can be due to a variety of factors, including advanced age, chronic illness, or sudden injury.

Other patients may experience a slower decline in their condition, with their health deteriorating over a longer period. This may be due to factors such as the nature of the patient's illness or the patient's overall health and resilience. Slow decline refers to a gradual deterioration in a patient's health over a period of weeks or months. This type of decline may be less sudden and distressing than a rapid decline, but it can still be difficult for the patient and their loved ones to cope with.

There are many factors that can contribute to a slow decline in a patient's health. Some common illnesses that can cause slow decline include:

- Chronic illnesses: Chronic illnesses such as heart disease, diabetes, or kidney disease can cause a slow decline in a patient's health as the condition progresses over time.

- Dementia: Dementia is a progressive brain disorder that can cause a slow decline in a patient's cognitive and physical abilities.

- COPD: Chronic obstructive pulmonary disease (COPD) is a lung condition that causes breathing difficulties and can cause a slow decline in a patient's respiratory function.

- HIV/AIDS: HIV/AIDS is a viral infection that attacks the immune system and can cause a slow decline in a patient's overall health.

Some patients may experience unexpected complications that significantly impact their condition. These complications may be related to the patient's illness or to unrelated medical issues.

There are many factors that can contribute to unexpected complications in a patient's health. Some common causes may include:

- Infections: Unexpected infections can occur in patients who are already seriously ill and can cause a rapid deterioration in their condition.

- Adverse reactions to medications: Some patients may experience unexpected side effects or allergic reactions to medications, which can impact their condition.

- Sudden medical emergencies: Patients may also experience unexpected medical emergencies, such as a heart attack or stroke, which can significantly impact their condition.

The hospice case manager must closely monitor the patient's condition and work with the patient and their family to manage any symptoms and provide the best possible care and support during this time. The hospice team should also be prepared to respond to any unexpected changes in the patient's condition and to provide appropriate treatment as needed.

Some patients may experience periods of stability, where their condition does not worsen significantly. This may be due to effective symptom management or the plateauing of the patient's illness. A stable trajectory refers to a period of time during which a patient's condition does not significantly worsen or improve. This may be a welcome respite for the patient and their loved ones, as it can provide some time to adjust to the patient's illness and make plans for the future.

There are several factors that can contribute to a stable trajectory for a patient. These may include:

- Effective symptom management: If the patient's symptoms are well-controlled, their condition may remain stable. This may be due to effective pain management, treatment of any underlying infections or other complications, and other supportive care measures.

- Plateauing of the illness: Some illnesses may reach a plateau or a point at which they are no longer progressing. This can result in a stable trajectory for the patient.

- Good overall health: A patient who is in generally good health may be more resilient and able to cope with their illness, which may result in a more stable trajectory.

An extended prognosis in hospice refers to a situation in which a patient's condition is expected to deteriorate slowly over a longer period of time, often several months or more. This can be a challenging situation for both the patient and their loved ones, as it can be difficult to predict how the patient's condition will progress and to make plans for the future.

It is possible for a patient to be revoked from hospice services due to an extended prognosis, although this is generally not common. Hospice care is designed for patients who are expected to have a prognosis of six months or less if their illness follows its normal course. However, some patients may experience an extended prognosis due to a variety of factors, such as the nature of their illness, their overall health and resilience, or the effectiveness of symptom management.

In these cases, the hospice team may continue to provide care and support to the patient if they continue to meet the criteria for hospice eligibility and if the patient and their family wish to continue receiving hospice services. However, if the patient's condition significantly improves or if they no longer meet the criteria for hospice eligibility, they may be revoked from hospice services.

It is important for the hospice team to regularly assess the patient's condition and to work with the patient and their family to determine the best course of care. The hospice team should also be prepared to help the patient and their family to transition to other forms of care if necessary.

In some cases, a patient may experience sudden death, which may be due to factors such as a sudden cardiac event or a severe complication related to the patient's illness. Sudden death refers to the unexpected and rapid loss of life, often within a matter of hours or days. This can be a shocking and distressing experience for the patient's loved ones, as they may not have had the opportunity to say goodbye or to make end-of-life plans.

There are many factors that can contribute to sudden death in a patient. Some common causes may include:

- Sudden cardiac event: A sudden cardiac event, such as a heart attack, can cause rapid and unexpected death.

- Severe complications: Some patients may experience severe complications related to their illness that can lead to sudden death. For example, a patient with advanced cancer may develop a blood clot or other serious complication that can cause a rapid deterioration in their condition.

- Accidents or injuries: Patients may also experience sudden death as a result of an accident or injury, such as a car crash or a fall.

The hospice team should always be prepared for the possibility of sudden death and be prepared to provide support and comfort to the patient's loved ones during this difficult time. The hospice team can also help the patient's loved ones to understand what happened and cope with their grief.

Case study: During her next visit, Sarah, Janice, and Tammy sat down in the living room of Mrs. Nesbitt's house. Janice and Tammy were visibly concerned, and Sarah could see the worry etched on their faces. Janice and Tammy asked Sarah about their mom's trajectory with her worsening COPD and CHF. They were worried about her prognosis and wanted to know what to expect in the coming days and weeks. Sarah understood the concerns of Janice and Tammy regarding their mother's prognosis and trajectory with her COPD and CHF. She acknowledged that this is a difficult time for them both and provided them with information and support as much as possible.

Sarah explained that as the diseases progress, symptoms such as shortness of breath, fatigue, and cough may become more severe, and Mrs. Nesbitt may become more dependent on others for care and may have more difficulty with activities of daily living. She also discussed that as the disease progresses, their mother may become increasingly fragile, and the likelihood of hospitalization or emergency department visits may increase. She also discussed that patients with advanced COPD and CHF may experience periods of rapid deterioration, where symptoms can worsen quickly.

Sarah also emphasized that each person's experience with COPD and CHF is unique, and that Mrs. Nesbitt's trajectory may not follow the typical pattern. She also emphasized that the hospice team is dedicated to providing the best possible care for Mrs. Nesbitt and will be closely monitoring her condition and adjusting the plan of care as needed.

Sarah provided information and support to Janice and Tammy about end-of-life care and the dying process. She discussed the importance of providing comfort and support to their mom during this time, and the importance of addressing their own emotional and spiritual needs as well. She also provided them with information about bereavement support services that are available to them after their mother's passing.

Sarah also provided Janice and Tammy with a guide on how to provide care for their mother during the final days, including caregiving tips, guidance on handling emotions and how to communicate with her in her state. She also provided contact information for the hospice team and encouraged them to reach out to the team if they have any questions or concerns. Sarah reminded them that Hospice is a team-based approach, and they will be there to support them throughout the process and that they should not hesitate to reach out to the team for any help.

Sarah then sent an encrypted email to update the rest of the hospice team about the current situation and the concerns of Janice and Tammy. She informed the team members of the changes in Mrs. Nesbitt's condition, and the support that Janice and Tammy required. She requested for the social worker, chaplain, and bereavement counselor to reach out to Mrs. Nesbitt and her family as well to provide additional support and guidance.

Signs of Imminent Death

One of the first signs of impending death is a change in the patient's breathing pattern. This can include shallow, irregular breathing, or periods of apnea (temporary cessation of breathing). The patient may also exhibit a decrease in their respiratory rate, or their breathing may become louder and more labored.

Another common sign of impending death is a change in the patient's skin color and temperature. The skin may become pale or mottled, and it may feel cool to the touch. The patient may also experience changes in their blood pressure, with a decrease in systolic blood pressure (the top number) and an increase in diastolic blood pressure (the bottom number).

As the body begins to shut down, the patient may also exhibit a decrease in their level of consciousness. They may become drowsy or unresponsive, and they may no longer respond to stimuli such as voices or touch.

In addition to these physical signs, the patient may also experience psychological and emotional changes. They may become anxious or agitated, or they may exhibit signs of delirium. The patient may also become withdrawn and less communicative.

It is important for the hospice nurse to closely monitor the patient for these signs and symptoms, and to provide support and comfort as needed. The nurse should also communicate with the patient's family and other members of the care team about any changes in the patient's condition and provide education and support to help them understand and prepare for the end of life. The nurse should also work closely with the patient's healthcare provider to ensure that the patient's pain and other symptoms are managed effectively.

The hospice case manager may need to provide end-of-life nursing care during their visits, such as wound care for terminal pressure ulcers, administering medications to control symptoms, or providing emotional support to the patient and their family. The nurse should always prioritize the patient's comfort and quality of life during this difficult time.

Performing thorough and regular assessments is an important aspect of a hospice case manager's role in caring for patients at the end of life. These assessments allow the case manager to gain a comprehensive understanding of the patient's current condition and needs, and to identify any changes that may have occurred since the last assessment. This information is essential for developing and adapting the patient's care plan, which may include physical, emotional, and social support, as well as addressing any practical needs related to the patient's living environment and support system.

During the assessment process, a hospice case manager may use a variety of tools and techniques, such as observations, interviews with the patient and their caregivers, and review of medical records. They may also consult with other members of the hospice team, such as doctors, nurses, social workers, and chaplains, to gather additional information and perspectives.

By performing regular assessments, a hospice case manager can help to ensure that patients receive the most appropriate and effective care and support and that any changes in their condition or needs are promptly addressed. This can greatly improve the patient's quality of life and end-of-life experience and provide peace of mind and comfort for the patient and their loved ones.

The role of the hospice nurse in the care of a patient who is nearing the end of life is to provide compassionate, supportive care that helps the patient and their family to prepare for and manage the end-of-life process. This care should be individualized to meet the needs of each patient and their family, and it should be provided with sensitivity, empathy, and professionalism. By providing support and guidance, and by working closely with the healthcare team and the patient's family, the hospice nurse can help to ensure that the patient experiences a peaceful and comfortable end of life.

Case study: During Sarah's visit, she noticed that Mrs. Nesbitt's condition had significantly worsened. She noticed that Mrs. Nesbitt was breathing more shallowly and rapidly and that her skin had taken on a bluish tinge. Mrs. Nesbitt's daughter Janice was present and asked Sarah what signs and symptoms she should be watching for as her mother approached the end of her life.

Sarah explained that as a person nears the end of their life, their breathing may become more shallow and rapid, their skin may take on a bluish tinge, and they may become less responsive to their surroundings. She also mentioned that other signs of approaching death may include a decreased need for food and fluids, drowsiness, confusion, and a decrease in blood pressure and heart rate.

Sarah also emphasized the importance of being present and providing comfort to Mrs. Nesbitt during this time. She also provided Janice with information on how to provide comfort measures such as positioning, skin care, and mouth care to ensure her mother's comfort as much as possible. She also provided Janice with information on how to administer medication to alleviate any discomfort or pain that Mrs. Nesbitt may be experiencing.

Sarah also explained that it is normal for the body to go through physical changes at the end of life, and that these changes should not be feared or feared but understood as a natural part of the dying process. She emphasized that it is important for Janice to be prepared for what to expect and to provide emotional support and comfort to her mother.

Chapter 5

Working with Facilities

Providing hospice care in nursing homes and other long-term care facilities is a common part of the role of the hospice case manager. These facilities often have a team of healthcare professionals, including nurses, aides, and therapists, who work together to provide care to residents. The hospice case manager is responsible for coordinating the hospice care provided by this team and ensuring that it is aligned with the goals and wishes of the patient.

One of the key responsibilities of the hospice case manager in a long-term care facility is to work closely with the facility staff to ensure that the patient's care plan is being followed. This may involve conducting assessments, providing symptom management and pain control, and coordinating with other members of the hospice care team, such as chaplains, social workers, and volunteers. The hospice case manager should also be available to answer questions and provide support to the facility staff as needed.

A typical facility visit for a hospice case manager might include conducting assessments of the patient, reviewing the care plan, coordinating with the facility staff and other members of the hospice care team, and communicating with the patient and their family. The hospice case manager needs to be organized and prepared for these visits, as there may be a lot of information to review and discuss.

There are several potential challenges that the hospice case manager may face when working in a long-term care facility. One challenge is ensuring that the patient's care is coordinated and consistent, particularly if the patient is being cared for by multiple healthcare professionals. Another challenge is managing the patient's symptoms and providing emotional and spiritual support to both the patient and their family. It may also be difficult to provide hospice care in a facility that is not fully equipped or prepared to support the patient's needs.

Memory care communities present a unique set of challenges for hospice care. Many residents in these communities have advanced dementia or other cognitive impairments, which can make communication and symptom management more difficult. It is important for the hospice case manager to be patient and understanding when working with these residents, and to use techniques such as nonverbal communication and music therapy to connect with them.

Despite the challenges, working with memory care residents can be a rewarding experience for the hospice case manager. These residents may not be able to communicate their needs or feelings in the same way as someone without cognitive impairments, but they can still benefit from the comfort and support provided by hospice care. The hospice case manager can make a positive impact in the lives of these residents and their families by providing compassionate, respectful care.

Case study: Sarah, the hospice case manager, received a call from Janice, the daughter of her patient Mrs. Nesbitt, who informed her that she had taken her mother to the emergency room for symptoms of a stroke. Sarah immediately contacted the hospice social worker, Madilynn, and the two of them met Janice at the emergency room. The ER physician confirmed that Mrs. Nesbitt had suffered a cerebrovascular accident (CVA) and her prognosis was poor. Sarah and Madilynn provided emotional support to Janice as she struggled with the news of her mother's deteriorating condition.

Janice expressed her concerns about being able to provide adequate medical care for her mother at home, and Sarah and Madilynn informed her that Mrs. Nesbitt could continue receiving hospice services in a skilled nursing facility (SNF). Janice asked about receiving hospice services in the hospital, but the ER physician stated that a general inpatient (GIP) hospice admission would not be recommended as Mrs. Nesbitt was stable and not likely to pass within the next 5 days, which is the time frame that Medicare has established for hospice to provide care in a hospital setting.

Sarah and Madilynn explained to Janice that in a SNF setting, hospice would continue to provide care to Mrs. Nesbitt, including symptom management and emotional support for both the patient and her family. They would also work closely with the SNF staff to ensure that Mrs. Nesbitt received appropriate care and that her pain and other symptoms were well-managed. Additionally, the hospice team would provide bereavement support for the family once Mrs. Nesbitt passed away.

Janice ultimately agreed to have her mother transferred to a local skilled nursing facility where she would continue to receive hospice services. Sarah and Madilynn assured Janice that they would continue to provide support and guidance throughout the process and that they would be available to her and her family whenever they needed.

The case manager will perform a *medication reconciliation* for their patient with each visit to their facility to ensure that the patient is receiving the correct medications at the correct dosages and that no refills are needed. This process involves reviewing the patient's current medications, comparing them to the medications that were previously prescribed, and identifying any discrepancies or potential issues.

To perform a medication reconciliation, the hospice case manager should work closely with the patient and their family, as well as other members of the hospice care team and the staff at the long-term care facility, to gather a complete list of the patient's medications. This may involve reviewing the patient's medication list with the patient and their family, as well as reviewing any available medical records or contacting the patient's other healthcare providers.

Once the hospice case manager has gathered a complete list of the patient's medications, they should compare this list to the medications that were previously prescribed to the patient. This may involve reviewing the patient's medication history, as well as consulting with other members of the hospice care team and the staff at the long-term care facility. The hospice case manager should look for discrepancies between the current and previous medication lists and should identify any potential issues, such as medication interactions or inappropriate dosing.

If the hospice case manager identifies any discrepancies or potential issues with the patient's medications, they should work with the patient, their family, and other members of the hospice care team, as well as the staff at the long-term care facility, to resolve these issues. This may involve consulting with the patient's primary care physician or other healthcare providers, as well as working with the pharmacy to ensure that the patient has the correct medications and is able to access them.

The hospice case manager will have a professional and collaborative relationship with the staff at the long-term care facility where their patient is receiving care. This includes working closely with the administrative staff, the nursing staff, the dietary staff, the housekeeping staff, the director of nursing, and even the concierge.

To establish a positive and professional relationship with the facility staff, the hospice case manager should communicate regularly with the staff about the patient's care. This may involve discussing the patient's care plan and any changes or updates to the plan, as well as addressing any concerns or issues that may arise.

The hospice case manager should also work closely with the facility staff to ensure that the patient is receiving the best possible care. This may involve coordinating with the staff to access resources and support for the patient, such as additional medical equipment or supplies.
In addition to communication and coordination, the hospice case manager should also be respectful and professional when interacting with the facility staff. This includes being punctual for meetings and appointments, following through on commitments, and being open to feedback and suggestions.

Overall, the relationship between the hospice case manager and the facility staff should be one of collaboration and mutual respect. By working together and communicating effectively, the hospice case manager and the facility staff can help to ensure that the patient receives the best possible care.

To provide the best possible care, the hospice case manager will establish and maintain relationships with key staff members at long-term care facilities. The following are some key staff members that the hospice case manager should talk to and work with during visits to their patients.

The facility *Administrator* or *Director* is responsible for managing the overall operations of the facility and ensuring that the patient's care needs are met. The hospice case manager should work closely with the nursing home administrator to ensure that the patient's care needs are being met and to address any issues that may arise. The hospice case manager should have a positive and professional relationship with the facility administrator at the long-term care facility where their patient is receiving care.

The *Director of Nursing (DON)*, or *Health Services Director*, at the long-term care facility is responsible for overseeing the nursing staff and the delivery of nursing care. The hospice case manager will work closely with the facility director of nursing and the *Assistant Director of Nursing (ADON)* to ensure that their patient is receiving the best possible care. This includes collaborating with the DON and ADON to develop and implement the patient's care plan, coordinating with the nursing staff to provide medical care, and communicating with the patient and their family about the patient's care.

To establish a positive and professional relationship with the clinical leadership, the hospice case manager should communicate regularly with them about the patient's care. This may involve discussing the patient's care plan and any changes or updates to the plan, as well as addressing any concerns or issues that may arise. The hospice case manager should also be open to feedback and suggestions from the DON and ADON and should be willing to work together to resolve any challenges that may arise in the patient's care.

> *Pro-Tip: It is often the director of nursing or the assistant director of nursing who will make the decision for which hospice provider to refer a patient to. Be a valuable resource for them.*

The *nursing* staff at the long-term care facility plays a crucial role in the patient's care and should be consulted with every visit to the facility. The hospice case manager will communicate with the nursing staff about the patient's care needs and coordinate with them to ensure that the patient's care is delivered in a timely and effective manner. The case manager may work with several nurses in each facility. It is best practice to get to know every nurse on every floor of a facility. This will make your job easier, as well as make it more natural for the facility to provide new patient referrals to your hospice provider.

In some assisted living facilities, *Medication Techs* or *Certified Residential Medication Aid (CRMAs)* may be utilized to assist with the administration of medications to residents. These individuals have received specialized training in medication administration and are responsible for helping to ensure that residents receive their medications as prescribed by their healthcare provider. They can often be relied on for information and support when nursing staff are not available or aren't staffed in a community.

The *caregiving* staff at the long-term care facility play a vital role in the patient's daily care and should be included in the hospice care plan. The hospice case manager should communicate with the caregiving staff about the patient's care needs and coordinate with them to ensure that the patient's care is delivered in a timely and effective manner.

The *dietary* staff at the long-term care facility are responsible for managing the patient's nutrition and hydration needs and should be included in the hospice care plan. This includes collaborating with the dietary staff to develop a plan for the patient's nutritional needs, coordinating with the nursing staff to monitor the patient's nutrition, and communicating with the patient and their family about the patient's nutritional status. The hospice case manager should work closely with the dietary staff to ensure that the patient is receiving appropriate nutrition and hydration and to address any issues that may arise.

The *housekeeping* staff at the long-term care facility are responsible for maintaining the cleanliness and safety of the patient's living environment. The hospice case manager should work with the housekeeping staff to ensure that the patient's living environment is safe and clean. The housekeeping staff is an important component of a patient's quality of life and the case manager should take time to get to know them.

The *concierge* or *receptionist* at the long-term care facility can provide valuable support and resources to the patient and their family, including assistance with transportation and appointments. The hospice case manager should work with the concierge to ensure that the patient and their family have knowledge of and access to the support and resources available to them.

The facility's *primary care physician* is responsible for managing the patient's overall medical care. The hospice case manager should work with the primary care physician to ensure that the patient's medical needs are being met and to coordinate the delivery of medical care. It is unlikely that an assisted living facility or stand-alone memory care community will have a primary care physician or even medical director. In this event, the hospice case manager will work with the patient's personal primary care provider or the facility visiting physician in some cases.

The hospice case manager also plays a key role in marketing the hospice to facilities and other potential referral sources. The Community Liaison is typically responsible for building relationships with referral sources and promoting the hospice to potential clients, but the hospice case manager can also contribute to this effort by providing information about the services and benefits of hospice care to facility staff and patients. The hospice case manager's role in building relationships with facilities and providing high-quality care can directly affect the success of the Community Liaison in attracting new clients.

General Inpatient or GIP hospice visits refer to hospice care provided in a hospital setting. A hospice provider may provide hospice services in a hospital for a variety of reasons, such as for patients who require more intensive medical care like intubation or for patients who have experienced a sudden decline in their condition. Some hospitals have hospice services that they provide in-house but may refer to hospice providers to provide support from time to time. Families may also wish to work with a specific hospice provider and will request to use their services in lieu of the hospital's hospice services.

One of the limitations of GIP hospice care is that it is typically provided for a limited period of time, typically no more than 5 days. This can be challenging for patients and their families, as it may not allow sufficient time for the hospice team to address all of the patient's needs.

To ensure that the patient receives the best possible care during a GIP hospice visit, the hospice case manager will need to coordinate closely with the hospital staff. This may involve working with the hospital's doctors, nurses, and other healthcare professionals to develop and implement the patient's care plan.

The hospice case manager should be a resource and support for facility staff and other members of the hospice care team. By providing education and training, as well as access to resources and support, the hospice case manager can help to ensure that the patient receives the highest quality of care possible. By working together, the hospice case manager and the facility staff can make a positive difference in the lives of the patients and families they serve.

Case Study: During Sarah's visit to the skilled nursing facility, she provided a variety of hospice services to Mrs. Nesbitt. She began by conducting a comprehensive assessment of Mrs. Nesbitt's physical, emotional, and social needs. This included taking vital signs, observing for any signs of discomfort or distress, and identifying any symptoms or concerns such as pain, shortness of breath, or fatigue.

Sarah also reviewed Mrs. Nesbitt's medications and made any necessary adjustments to her plan of care. She provided education to the nursing staff on how to administer comfort measures and symptom management medications including indications for use and contraindications. She also provided emotional support to Janice and her sister Tammy and made referrals to the hospice chaplain and social worker.

Sarah met with the Director of Nursing and the Administrator of the facility to discuss and coordinate Mrs. Nesbitt's care with the facility staff. She shared the patient's care plan and discussed any specific needs or concerns that the facility staff should be aware of. Sarah also made sure that the facility staff were trained on how to provide the specific hospice care needs for Mrs. Nesbitt. They discussed ways to improve the coordination of hospice care for Mrs. Nesbitt and other hospice patients in the facility.

One suggestion was for Sarah to provide in-services for the facility staff on topics such as symptom management, end-of-life care, and advanced care planning. An *in-service* refers to a training session provided by a professional, such as Sarah, to educate and update the knowledge and skills of the facility staff on a specific topic related to their field of work. Sarah and the hospice team worked with the facility staff to schedule these in-services, which helped ensure that all facility staff members were up to date on the latest information and best practices for caring for hospice patients.

During her visit, Sarah also interacted with different facility staff such as the nursing staff, the physical therapist, and the occupational therapist. She provided guidance on how to assist Mrs. Nesbitt with activities of daily living and any other specific needs. Sarah also discussed any updates on Mrs. Nesbitt's condition and made any necessary changes to her care plan. By working closely with the facility staff, Sarah was able to ensure that Mrs. Nesbitt received the highest quality of hospice care while staying in the skilled nursing facility.

Chapter 6

The Death Visit

Hospice care is focused on improving the quality of life for patients who are facing a terminal illness. While death visits are an important part of the hospice nurse's role, they typically spend much more of their time providing care and support to patients to help them live as comfortably as possible in their final stages of life.

This may involve providing symptom management and pain control, assisting with activities of daily living, and providing emotional and spiritual support to the patient and their family. The hospice nurse may also work closely with other members of the hospice care team, such as doctors, social workers, and chaplains, to coordinate the patient's care and address any needs or concerns that may arise.

In addition to providing direct care to patients, the hospice nurse may also spend time working with the patient's family and caregivers to provide education and support. This may involve helping the family understand the patient's diagnosis and prognosis, as well as providing guidance on how to manage the patient's symptoms and provide care at home.

Overall, the hospice nurse's focus is on helping patients live their remaining time as comfortably and meaningfully as possible, and death visits are just one aspect of the case manager's workload.

However, the *death visit* is an important part of the hospice care process, and it is a time when the hospice case manager plays a critical role in supporting the patient's family. The death visit is a time for the family to say goodbye to their loved one and begin the grieving process. It is also a time for the hospice case manager to provide emotional and spiritual support to the family and to ensure that their needs are met during this difficult time. If a patient's death occurs in a facility, the hospice nurse may be called on to provide emotional support to staff, particularly if the patient was a resident for a long time. No matter the setting, whether in the home or a facility, the hospice nurse will approach their patient's death with compassion and professionalism.

The hospice case manager is responsible for *pronouncing the death* of the patient. This is a formal process that involves checking for clinical signs of death and documenting the time of death. In the absence of the hospice case manager, a facility RN may pronounce the death of a patient, provided they follow the facility or hospice procedures and document all relevant times and pertinent information needed to thoroughly document the death. Clinical signs of death include the cessation of breathing and the absence of a pulse. The hospice case manager may also check for signs of *rigor mortis*, which is the stiffening of the muscles that occurs after death.

The *stages of death* are a series of physical and emotional changes that a person may experience as they near the end of their life. Understanding these stages can help hospice case managers provide compassionate care and support for their patients and their families. The generally accepted stages of death include pre-active dying; active dying; final stages or imminent death; dying process or death; and after death. Many hospices will combine the active dying stage, final stage, and dying process stage to simply: active dying, which usually includes when a person's death is imminent.

One of the earliest stages of death is *pre-active dying*. During this stage, the person may experience a decline in physical and mental functioning and may have difficulty eating, drinking, and communicating. They may also have trouble sleeping and may experience confusion or delirium. As a hospice case manager, it's important to be attuned to these changes and to provide support and comfort as needed. A person may be in the pre-active stage for days, weeks, or even months.

The next stage is *active dying*, which typically lasts for three to seven days. During this stage, the person's body begins to shut down and they may become more withdrawn and less responsive. They may also experience respiratory changes, such as shortness of breath and congestion. The hospice case managers will monitor the person's vital signs and provide palliative care, including pain management and comfort measures.

As the person approaches the final stages of death, they may experience a range of physical and emotional changes. They may become unconscious or unresponsive, and their breathing may become shallow or irregular. They may also experience muscle spasms or twitching. It's important for hospice case managers to provide comfort and support during this time, and to be present for the person and their family.

A patient may *"rally"* when their condition improves temporarily after a period of decline. This can be a physically and emotionally challenging time for both the patient and their loved ones.

From a physiological perspective, a rally may involve an improvement in the patient's vital signs and overall functioning. For example, they may have more energy, be able to eat and drink more, and have fewer symptoms such as pain or shortness of breath.

However, it is important to understand that a rally does not necessarily mean that the patient will live longer. It may simply be a temporary improvement that is followed by a return to decline. It is also important to recognize that a rally can be emotionally challenging for the patient and their loved ones, as it can raise hopes and expectations that may not be realistic.

In the event of a patient rally, it is important for the hospice nurse to closely monitor the patient's condition and communicate with the healthcare team to determine the best course of action. The caregiver should also be supportive and understanding and be prepared for the possibility of a return to decline. It may be helpful for the caregiver to have open and honest conversations with the hospice nurse and other members of the healthcare team about the patient's prognosis and treatment goals.

One of the final stages of death is the *dying process*, which can last for several hours or days. During this time, the person's body continues to shut down, and they may experience a range of physical and emotional changes. They may have difficulty breathing and may experience changes in their skin color and temperature. They may also have hallucinations or delirium. It's important for hospice case managers to be aware of these cognitive changes so they can support the patient and their family and help them make sense of the patients changing behaviors.

Before pronouncing a death, it's important to confirm that the person has indeed passed away. This can be done by checking for signs of life, such as a pulse, breathing, or responsiveness. To do this, the healthcare professional will typically listen for heart and lung sounds using a stethoscope for 2 minutes, watching for any rise and fall of the patient's chest, and taking distal pulses. In general, the absence of a pulse or heartbeat and the absence of lung sounds are both strong indicators that the person has passed away. However, it's important to note that it's possible for heart and lung sounds to be present for a short period of time after the person has passed away, so the hospice nurse will continue to continue to monitor the person for at least several minutes to confirm their passing.

The final stage of death is the period of time after the person has passed away. During this time, it's important for hospice case managers to support the family and to ensure that all necessary arrangements are made. This may include coordinating with funeral homes, preparing death certificates, and providing bereavement support.

After a patient has passed away, the nurse is responsible for preparing the body for transfer to the funeral home or for burial or cremation. This process is often referred to as *"caring for the deceased."*

First, the nurse will remove any tubes, medical equipment, or jewelry that may have been in use during the patient's final hours. This may include oxygen masks, IV lines, and catheters. The nurse will then gently clean the body, taking care to preserve the dignity and respect of the deceased.

The nurse may also gently close the patient's eyes and mouth and may arrange the arms and legs in a natural position. The nurse may also cover the body with a sheet or other cloth, depending on the preferences of the patient and their family.

The nurse will then make arrangements for the body to be transferred to the funeral home or other location as directed by the patient's family or advanced directives. This may involve coordinating with the funeral home or other transfer service and may also involve obtaining necessary documentation or permissions.

It is important for the nurse to be compassionate and understanding during this process, and to work closely with the patient's family to ensure that their wishes are respected and carried out. The nurse is also responsible for providing emotional support to the family during this difficult time.

After the patient's death, the hospice case manager has several tasks to complete. Depending on the hospice agency or local laws, these may include:

- Notifying the patient's primary care physician and any other relevant healthcare professionals of the death. This may include notifying the county medical examiner in some jurisdictions or situations.

- Contacting the patient's next of kin or designated caregiver to inform them of the death and to provide support during the grieving process.

- Coordinating the transfer of the patient's body to the patient's chosen funeral home. This will involve calling the funeral home to inform them of the patient's passing and waiting with the patient's body until they arrive.

- Arranging for any necessary funeral or cremation services, in consultation with the patient's family.

- Providing bereavement support to the patient's family. This may include connecting the family with grief counseling resources or providing them with information on how to cope with their loss.

- Documenting the patient's care and the circumstances of their death in the patient's medical record. This documentation should be thorough and accurate, as it will be used to inform future care decisions and to help with quality improvement efforts.

- Debriefing with the hospice care team to reflect on the patient's care and the circumstances of their death. This can help the team to learn from the experience and to improve their care in the future.

- Reviewing the patient's care plan and updating it as needed. This may include revising the patient's goals and objectives or modifying their treatment plan.

The death visit is a difficult and emotional time for the patient's family and the hospice care team. It is important for the hospice case manager to handle this event with compassion, professionalism, and sensitivity, and to provide the necessary support and guidance to help the family through this difficult time.

As a hospice nurse, it is natural to have complicated feelings about death and dying, as it is a deeply personal and emotional experience for both the patient and their loved ones. It is important for hospice nurses to acknowledge and reconcile their own feelings about death and dying, as it can help them to better care for their patients and families.

One way for hospice nurses to manage their feelings about death and dying is to recognize their own mortality. Acknowledging that death is a natural part of life can help to put things into perspective and provide a sense of acceptance. It can also be helpful for hospice nurses to reflect on their own values and beliefs about death and dying, as this can help them to better understand and support their patients and families.

Managing end-of-life care for others can also bring up complicated emotions, such as sadness, grief, and even anger. It is important for hospice nurses to be aware of their own emotions and to find healthy ways to cope with them. This can include seeking support from colleagues, participating in self-care activities, and seeking counseling or therapy if needed.

During the death visit, hospice nurses may also experience a range of emotions. It can be helpful for them to practice self-compassion and allow themselves to feel their emotions, while also remembering that they are there to provide support and comfort to the patient and their family. It can also be helpful to debrief with a colleague or supervisor after the death visit, as this can provide an opportunity to process and reflect on the experience.

Case study: As hospice nurse Sarah arrived at the nursing home, she was greeted by Janice and Tammy, the daughters of her patient, Mrs. Nesbitt. Sarah had been working closely with the nursing staff over the last two weeks, as Mrs. Nesbitt's condition had been rapidly deteriorating. Sarah knew that the end was near and had made the decision to increase the frequency of her visits from every other day to daily, in order to provide the best possible care for Mrs. Nesbitt and support for her family. As Sarah entered the room, she immediately noticed the signs and symptoms of imminent death. Sarah approached the bedside, where Mrs. Nesbitt lay peacefully, and took her hand, offering words of comfort and reassurance to both Mrs. Nesbitt and her daughters.

Sarah, upon noticing the physical signs of imminent death in Mrs. Nesbitt, began to take necessary steps to ensure that the passing of Mrs. Nesbitt was as comfortable as possible for both her and her family. One of the first things Sarah did was to ask the facility dietary staff to prepare a hospitality tray for Mrs. Nesbitt's family. The tray included a variety of light snacks and beverages for the family to have during their time at the bedside. Sarah explained to the family that this was a small way for the hospice team and the facility to support them during this difficult time and that they were welcome to enjoy the tray at any time.

During her visit, Sarah observed that Mrs. Nesbitt had become increasingly unresponsive, and her vital signs were indicating that death was imminent. She immediately notified the nursing staff and contacted the rest of the hospice team, including the bereavement counselor and chaplain, to come to the facility. Sarah provided emotional support to Janice and Tammy, explaining what signs and symptoms to expect and helping them understand the process of dying. She also made sure that Mrs. Nesbitt was comfortable and free of pain by administering medications from the comfort kit as needed.

Sarah noticed that Mrs. Nesbitt's breathing had become shallow and irregular, and her skin had taken on a mottled, purplish hue. Her pulse was weak and thready, and her blood pressure had dropped significantly. These were all physical signs that Mrs. Nesbitt was nearing the end of her life. Sarah knew that it was important to provide comfort and support to both Mrs. Nesbitt and her family during this difficult time. She made sure to keep the room quiet and peaceful, and to speak softly and calmly to Mrs. Nesbitt and her daughters.

Sarah approached Mrs. Nesbitt's bedside and observed her for several minutes, noting that she had become unresponsive and had no signs of life. She checked for a pulse, and finding none, she listened for breath sounds and confirmed that Mrs. Nesbitt had passed away. Sarah followed proper protocol by waiting for two minutes to ensure that there were no signs of life before pronouncing the time of death. She then informed the nursing staff and Mrs. Nesbitt's family of her passing, offering her condolences and emotional support.

Once Mrs. Nesbitt passed away, Sarah completed the necessary tasks such as caring for the body and notifying the physician. She also provided bereavement support to Janice and Tammy, offering resources and information on how to cope with the loss of their mother. Sarah also contacted the nursing home administrator and the funeral home to make arrangements for Mrs. Nesbitt's body to be transported.

Sarah also worked with the hospice community liaison, Theresa, to schedule a debriefing meeting with the nursing home staff to provide support and education on end-of-life care. She also met with the Director of Nursing and the Administrator to discuss the care provided to Mrs. Nesbitt and identify any areas for improvement in the future. Throughout the process, Sarah maintained open communication with the nursing staff and other members of the hospice team to ensure that Mrs. Nesbitt received the best possible care during her final days.

Chapter 7

Documentation and Legal Issues

Accurate and thorough documentation is essential for the work of the hospice case manager. Not only does it help to ensure the best possible care for patients and their families, but it also protects the hospice and the case manager from potential legal and ethical issues. In this chapter, we will explore the importance of documentation, legal and ethical considerations in hospice care, and how to maintain confidentiality and HIPAA compliance.

As a hospice case manager, you will be responsible for maintaining detailed and accurate records of the care you provide to patients and their families. This will include everything from initial assessments and care plans to daily notes and updates on patients' conditions and progress. This documentation is crucial for ensuring that patients receive the right treatments and support and that they are making progress toward their goals.

In addition to the practical benefits of documentation, it is also important for legal and ethical reasons. In the event of a legal dispute or complaint, detailed and accurate documentation can provide important evidence to support your actions and decisions. It can also help to protect you from potential accusations of negligence or misconduct.

There are also a number of legal and ethical considerations that the hospice case manager must be aware of. These include issues related to informed consent, end-of-life decisions, and maintaining patients' dignity and autonomy.

There are several consent forms that the hospice case manager or liaison may need to obtain from the patient or their Power of Attorney when admitting a patient to hospice. These forms are designed to ensure that the patient's wishes are respected and that their rights are protected.

One important form is the *hospice election form*, which is signed by the patient (or their Power of Attorney) to confirm that they are electing to receive hospice care. This form should be signed as soon as possible after the patient is admitted to hospice and should be kept in the patient's medical record.

The hospice election form is a legally binding document that is used to confirm a patient's decision to enroll in hospice care. The form is used to provide information about the patient's medical condition and prognosis, as well as their treatment preferences and goals.

The hospice election form typically requests information about the patient's diagnosis, symptoms, and overall health status. It may also ask about the patient's treatment preferences, such as whether they wish to receive curative or palliative treatment. Additionally, the form may ask about the patient's goals for their end-of-life care, such as whether they wish to receive care at home or in a hospice facility.

The hospice election form is an important tool for ensuring that the patient's wishes are respected and that their care is aligned with their goals. It is typically used by the hospice case manager and other members of the hospice care team to develop the patient's care plan and to coordinate the delivery of care. The form may also be used by the hospice agency or other healthcare providers to track the patient's progress and to ensure that the patient's care meets the standards set by regulatory agencies.

Another important form is the *consent for treatment form*, which is signed by the patient (or their Power of Attorney) to give consent for the hospice team to provide care. This form should be signed as soon as possible after the patient is admitted to hospice and should be kept in the patient's medical record.

One of the key legal and ethical considerations in hospice care is *informed consent*. This refers to the process of ensuring that patients and their families are fully informed about their care options and that they understand the potential risks and benefits of each option. As a hospice case manager, you will be responsible for providing patients and their families with clear and concise information about their care options, and for helping them to make informed decisions about their treatment.

The purpose of the consent for treatment form is to ensure that the patient understands the nature of their illness, the treatment options available to them, and the potential risks and benefits of each option. The form also outlines the patient's right to refuse treatment or to change their treatment plan at any time.

The consent for treatment form should be signed by the patient or their legal guardian and should be kept on file with the hospice provider. The information on the form is used by the hospice team to develop the patient's care plan and to ensure that their care is consistent with their preferences and goals.

It is important for the hospice case manager to review the hospice election form and the consent for treatment form with the patient and their family, and to answer any questions they may have. This will help ensure that the patient fully understands their rights and responsibilities and that their treatment is consistent with their wishes.

The hospice team will also need to complete a comprehensive assessment of the patient's medical, social, and spiritual needs. This assessment should be completed as soon as possible after the patient is admitted to hospice and should be used to develop the patient's care plan. The care plan should be reviewed and updated regularly to ensure that it continues to meet the patient's needs.

In addition to these forms, the hospice team will also need to complete other documentation, such as medication lists, nursing notes, and physician orders. These documents should be kept in the patient's medical record and should be reviewed and updated regularly to ensure that they reflect the patient's current condition and care needs.

There are several legal considerations to keep in mind when completing documentation for hospice. It is important to ensure that all forms are signed by the appropriate parties and that the patient's rights and preferences are respected. It is also important to ensure that the patient's medical record is kept confidential and is only accessed by those who have a legitimate need to see it.

Another important legal and ethical consideration is end-of-life decision-making. In some cases, patients and their families may need to make difficult decisions about life-sustaining treatments, such as mechanical ventilation or feeding tubes. As a hospice case manager, you will need to help patients and their families understand their options and support them in making decisions that are in line with their values and preferences.

In addition to informed consent and end-of-life decision-making, it is also important for hospice case managers to maintain patients' dignity and autonomy. This means respecting patients' right to make decisions about their own care and supporting them in maintaining their independence and control over their lives. This can involve providing emotional and spiritual support, as well as helping patients to access resources and services that can improve their quality of life. This also means respecting a patient's decision to revoke hospice services.

The process of *revocation* from hospice services occurs when a patient decides to end their hospice care and return to traditional medical treatment. There are several reasons why a patient might choose to revoke hospice services. Some patients may feel that their condition has improved and they are no longer in need of hospice care. Others may wish to explore additional treatment options that are not available through hospice care.

There are also situations in which a patient might be revoked from hospice services. For example, if a patient's condition significantly improves and they are no longer eligible for hospice care, they may be revoked from the program. Additionally, if a patient is not following the care plan or is not receiving the necessary level of care, they may be revoked from hospice services.

In either case, the process of revocation typically involves the patient or their designated representative (such as a Power of Attorney) completing a revocation form, which is then reviewed by the hospice team. If the revocation is approved, the patient's hospice care will be terminated, and they will transition back to traditional medical treatment. It is important to note that revocation from hospice services is a rare occurrence, as most patients and their families find significant value in the comprehensive and supportive care provided by hospice.

There are also a number of important regulations and guidelines that the hospice case manager must be aware of. These include federal laws such as the Health Insurance Portability and Accountability Act (HIPAA), as well as professional standards and guidelines set by organizations such as the National Hospice and Palliative Care Organization (NHPCO).

HIPAA is a federal law that protects the privacy of a patient's health information. It sets out strict rules and regulations for how patient information can be collected, used, and disclosed, and imposes penalties for non-compliance. As a hospice case manager, you will need to be familiar with HIPAA and how it applies to your work, and to take steps to ensure that you are complying with the law.

To maintain confidentiality and HIPAA compliance, it is important to take a few key steps. First, make sure that you use secure and encrypted systems for storing and accessing patient records. This will help to prevent unauthorized access to sensitive information. Second, be careful about whom you share patient information with, and always get permission from patients or their authorized representatives before sharing any sensitive information. Finally, make sure that you follow all relevant laws and regulations regarding the protection of patient information.

The NHPCO is a professional organization that provides guidance and support to hospice and palliative care providers. It has developed a set of professional standards and guidelines that outline the key principles and practices of hospice care. As a hospice case manager, you will need to be familiar with these standards and guidelines and use them as a framework for your work.

In addition to federal laws and professional standards, there may also be state or local regulations that apply to hospice care. These can include licensing and certification requirements, as well as specific rules and guidelines for the provision of hospice services. As a hospice case manager, you will need to be aware of any relevant state or local regulations and ensure that you are complying with them.

Chapter 8

Working with Special Populations

As a hospice case manager, you will be working with patients and families who are facing a wide range of challenges and needs. This may include older adults, terminally ill children, and patients with advanced *dementia* and other cognitive impairments. In this chapter, we will explore some of the key considerations for working with these special populations, and how to provide the best possible care and support.

One of the special populations that hospice case managers may work with is older adults. Providing hospice care to older adults can be a rewarding and challenging experience for hospice nurses. As people age, they may be more prone to certain health issues and may have more complex care needs. Geriatric hospice care requires a specialized approach that takes into account the unique needs of older adults and their families.

As the population ages, the number of older adults who are eligible for hospice care is increasing. The "*Silver Tsunami*" refers to the large aging population of baby boomers in the United States and the potential impact this will have on healthcare and other industries. As baby boomers age and become more likely to require hospice care, there is concern about the ability of the healthcare system to meet the increased demand for hospice services.

One challenge of the Silver Tsunami is that it may lead to a shortage of healthcare professionals, including hospice nurses, to care for the aging population. This could lead to longer wait times for hospice services, as well as increased workload and stress for hospice nurses who are already stretched thin.

Another challenge is that many baby boomers are living with chronic illnesses that may require more complex and specialized care. Providing hospice care to older adults with multiple chronic conditions can be challenging and may require additional resources and support. These patients may have a variety of medical conditions, such as heart disease, cancer, or chronic obstructive pulmonary disease (COPD). They may also have cognitive impairments, such as dementia or Alzheimer's disease.

When working with older adults, it is important to be sensitive to their unique needs and challenges. This may include providing support for physical symptoms, such as pain or shortness of breath, as well as addressing psychological and social needs. It may also involve working with family members and caregivers to provide support and education.

Another challenge of geriatric hospice care is helping patients and their families navigate the end-of-life process. This may involve providing emotional and spiritual support, coordinating care with other members of the hospice team, and assisting with decision-making about care preferences. The hospice nurse should be prepared to provide this support in a compassionate and respectful manner, taking into account the patient's and family's cultural and spiritual beliefs.

Despite these challenges, providing hospice care to older adults can be a deeply rewarding experience for hospice nurses. By focusing on improving the quality of life for seniors nearing the end of their lives, hospice nurses can make a meaningful difference in the lives of their patients and their families. This can be a source of great job satisfaction for hospice nurses and can be a rewarding career path for those who are passionate about geriatric care.

Another special population that hospice case managers may work with is terminally ill children and their families. This can be a particularly challenging and emotional area of work, as it involves supporting families during some of the most difficult times in their lives.

Providing hospice care to terminally ill children and young people presents unique challenges and rewards for hospice professionals. The physical, emotional, and developmental needs of children and young people are different from those of adults, and hospice care must be tailored to meet these specific needs.

One of the main challenges of providing hospice care to children and young people is the need to support the entire family, not just the patient. Children and young people are often accompanied by parents, siblings, and other family members, who may be experiencing their own grief and stress. The hospice team must be prepared to provide support and guidance to all family members, not just the patient.

Another challenge is communicating with young patients about their illness and treatment options. Children may have a difficult time understanding their diagnosis and prognosis and may need additional support and explanation from the hospice team. It may also be challenging to engage children and young people in decision-making about their care, as they may not have the same level of understanding or autonomy as adults.

One of the key benefits of hospice care for children and young people is the opportunity to receive care in a home-like setting. Children and young people often feel more comfortable and at ease in familiar surroundings, and hospice care allows them to receive medical care and support in their own home or the home of a family member. This can help to reduce anxiety and stress for the patient and their family and can improve the overall quality of care.

Another benefit of hospice care for children and young people is the focus on symptom management and pain control. Children and young people may experience different symptoms and may have different reactions to medications than adults. Pain is a common symptom that children with terminal illnesses may experience, and effective pain management is essential to improving their quality of life. Hospice nurses are trained to provide pain management using a variety of approaches, including medication, relaxation techniques, and other non-pharmacological methods.

One of the main benefits of receiving pain control from a hospice nurse is that it can help children feel more comfortable and at ease. When a child is experiencing pain, it can be difficult for them to relax and enjoy activities, which can significantly impact their quality of life. By providing effective pain management, hospice nurses can help children feel more comfortable and able to participate in activities they enjoy.

Hospice nurses are also skilled in assessing and monitoring children's pain levels, which is essential for ensuring that pain management is effective. They can work with the child's primary care team to develop a comprehensive pain management plan that addresses the child's specific needs and preferences.

Another special population that hospice case managers may work with is patients with advanced dementia and other cognitive impairments. Providing hospice care to patients with advanced dementia and other cognitive impairments can be a challenging but rewarding experience for hospice nurses. These patients may have difficulty communicating their needs and may be unable to understand their diagnosis or the purpose of their treatment. As a result, it is important for the hospice nurse to meet the patient where they are at, mentally, and to focus on providing comfort and support rather than trying to reorient the patient to our reality.

One of the main challenges of providing hospice care to patients with cognitive impairment is managing pain. These patients may be unable to communicate their pain or may have difficulty understanding what is happening to them. As a result, it is important for the hospice nurse to use a variety of pain assessment tools and techniques, including nonverbal methods such as facial expressions and behavior, to identify and treat pain in these patients.

The PAINAD tool (Pain Assessment in Advanced Dementia) is a validated assessment tool that is used to assess pain in non-verbal patients, including those with advanced dementia. It is designed to be used by healthcare professionals who are trained in its use, such as hospice nurses.

The PAINAD tool consists of a series of behaviors that are commonly associated with pain, including facial expressions, vocalizations, and body movements. The healthcare professional assesses the patient's behavior using these criteria and scores the patient based on the severity of the behaviors observed. The scores are then used to guide the development of a pain management plan for the patient.

One of the benefits of using the PAINAD tool is that it can help to identify pain in patients who are unable to communicate their pain in other ways. This is particularly important in hospice care, where the focus is on providing symptom management and improving quality of life for the patient. By identifying and treating pain, the hospice nurse can help to improve the patient's comfort and reduce their suffering.

There are some limitations to the use of the PAINAD tool, however. It is not always accurate, and there may be other factors that contribute to the behaviors observed. In addition, it is important to consider the patient's overall clinical status and to use other assessment tools, such as the Brief Pain Inventory, as needed to ensure that the patient's pain is being managed effectively.

Another benefit, and challenge, of providing hospice care to patients with cognitive impairment is working with memory care communities. These communities often have specialized staff trained to care for patients with dementia and other cognitive impairments, and it is important for the hospice nurse to collaborate with this staff to ensure that the patient's care is coordinated and consistent.

The hospice nurse may also need to use nonverbal communication techniques and other strategies, such as music therapy, to connect with these patients and provide emotional and spiritual support. The hospice nurse will work with facility staff to obtain information about the patient's current condition and evaluate their plan of care. Working with memory care communities can be a very rewarding experience when the hospice nurse is knowledgeable about the complexities of caring for patients with dementia and coordinates their care with facility staff.

Working with the families of hospice patients with cognitive impairment can also be challenging. These families may have difficulty understanding the patient's condition and may need support and guidance as they navigate the complex and emotional process of end-of-life care. The hospice nurse should be available to provide information, support, and guidance to the patient's family, and should work closely with them to develop a care plan that meets the patient's needs and preferences.

There are several types of dementia that can affect hospice patients, including Alzheimer's disease, vascular dementia, and Lewy body dementia. Each type of dementia has its own unique challenges and characteristics, and it is important for the hospice nurse to understand these differences in order to provide the best possible care for the patient. For example, patients with Alzheimer's disease may experience memory loss, confusion, and changes in behavior, while patients with vascular dementia may experience problems with decision-making and planning. The hospice nurse should be familiar with these challenges and should work with the patient and their family to develop a care plan that addresses the patient's specific needs and preferences.

Alzheimer's disease is a progressive and degenerative brain disorder that is characterized by the gradual loss of memory and cognitive function. It is the most common cause of dementia in older adults and is characterized by the accumulation of abnormal proteins in the brain, which leads to the death of brain cells. There is no known cure for Alzheimer's disease, and treatment is focused on managing symptoms and slowing the progression of the disease.

The exact cause of Alzheimer's disease is not fully understood, but it is thought to be related to a combination of genetic, environmental, and lifestyle factors. Some people may be at higher risk of developing Alzheimer's disease due to genetic factors, while others may be more likely to develop the disease due to unhealthy lifestyle habits or exposure to certain environmental toxins.

There are several treatments available for Alzheimer's disease, including medications that can help to improve cognitive function and manage symptoms such as memory loss and confusion. These medications can be effective in slowing the progression of the disease, but they do not cure it. Other treatments for Alzheimer's disease may include non-pharmacological approaches, such as cognitive-behavioral therapy and other types of therapy, as well as support for caregivers and other forms of social support.

Vascular dementia is a type of cognitive impairment that results from reduced blood flow to the brain. This reduced blood flow can be caused by a variety of factors, including stroke, heart disease, and uncontrolled high blood pressure. When the brain does not receive enough oxygen and nutrients from the blood, it can become damaged, leading to the development of vascular dementia.

Vascular dementia is typically characterized by problems with memory, thinking, and decision-making abilities. It may also cause problems with language, visual-spatial abilities, and other cognitive functions. The severity of these symptoms can vary widely, depending on the underlying cause of the reduced blood flow and the extent of brain damage.

In some cases, vascular dementia can be treated or slowed with medications, lifestyle changes, and other interventions. For example, medications that control high blood pressure or lower cholesterol may be used to reduce the risk of further brain damage. Lifestyle changes, such as quitting smoking, eating a healthy diet, and getting regular exercise, can also help to prevent or manage vascular dementia.

While there is no cure for vascular dementia, there are many ways in which patients and their families can manage the condition and improve their quality of life. This may include working with a healthcare team to develop a care plan, using assistive devices or technologies to help with daily tasks, and seeking support from caregivers and other resources.

Lewy body dementia is a type of progressive cognitive impairment characterized by the accumulation of abnormal proteins called alpha-synuclein in the brain. It is the second most common form of dementia after Alzheimer's disease and is often misdiagnosed or overlooked due to the wide range of symptoms it can cause.

Symptoms of Lewy body dementia can include cognitive changes such as memory loss, confusion, and difficulty with decision-making, as well as movement changes such as tremors and rigidity, and behavioral changes such as hallucinations, delusions, and mood swings. The disease can also cause sleep disturbances and changes in autonomic functions such as blood pressure regulation and digestion.

Providing hospice care for patients with Lewy body dementia can be challenging due to the wide range of symptoms and the potential for rapid changes in the patient's condition. It is important for the hospice nurse to be proactive and vigilant in monitoring the patient's symptoms and adjusting their care plan as needed. This may involve working closely with the patient's primary care physician and other members of the hospice care team to manage medications, control symptoms, and provide emotional and spiritual support.

One of the unique challenges of caring for patients with Lewy body dementia is managing the patient's hallucinations and delusions. These symptoms can be distressing for the patient and may cause them to become agitated or confused. It is important for the hospice nurse to remain calm and reassuring when interacting with the patient and to try to redirect their attention to more positive or calming activities.

Another challenge of caring for patients with Lewy body dementia is managing their sleep disturbances. Patients with this type of dementia may experience difficulty falling asleep, staying asleep, or waking up at inappropriate times. This can lead to fatigue, confusion, and increased agitation. The hospice nurse may need to work with the patient and their family to develop strategies for improving sleep, such as creating a consistent sleep routine, avoiding caffeine and alcohol, and using relaxation techniques.

Overall, providing hospice care for patients with Lewy body dementia requires a high level of compassion, patience, and skill. By working closely with the patient and their family, the hospice nurse can help to improve the patient's quality of life and provide support during a difficult time.

It is important to note that dementia is not a normal part of aging and can be caused by various factors, including genetics, head injuries, and certain medical conditions. While there is currently no cure for dementia, there are ways to manage the condition and improve the quality of life for individuals living with dementia.

Working with special populations is an important part of the work of the hospice case manager. By being sensitive to the unique needs and challenges of each population, and by providing care that is tailored to their individual circumstances, the hospice case manager can make a positive difference in the lives of terminally ill patients and their families.

Chapter 9

Advanced Care Planning

As a hospice case manager, you will be working with patients and their families to help them plan for end-of-life care. This may include discussing patients' end-of-life wishes, making decisions about life-sustaining treatments, and providing bereavement support after a patient's death. In this chapter, we will explore some of the key considerations for advanced care planning, and how to provide the best possible support and guidance to patients and their families.

As a key member of the hospice care team, the hospice case manager plays a crucial role in helping patients and their families navigate the end-of-life process. One of the most important aspects of this role is facilitating discussions about end-of-life wishes and preferences. These discussions should involve not only the patient, but also their family and other members of the hospice care team, as appropriate.

The hospice case manager should work with the patient and their family to help them understand their treatment options and the potential risks and benefits of each option. This may include discussing the use of palliative care, which is designed to alleviate symptoms and improve the patient's quality of life, as well as the use of hospice care, which focuses on providing comfort and support for patients who are expected to have six months or less to live.

As a hospice nurse, it's important to understand the difference between palliative care and hospice care. *Palliative care* is a type of medical care that focuses on relieving symptoms and improving the quality of life for patients with serious illnesses. It can be provided at any stage of an illness and is often provided alongside curative treatment.

Hospice care, on the other hand, is a type of palliative care that is specifically designed for patients who are in the final stages of a terminal illness and are no longer seeking curative treatment. Hospice care focuses on providing comfort and support to patients and their families and aims to help patients live their remaining time as comfortably and meaningfully as possible.

In addition to discussing treatment options, the hospice case manager should also help the patient and their family understand their rights and preferences when it comes to end-of-life care. This may involve discussing the use of advanced directives, such as living wills and durable power of attorney for healthcare, which allow patients to document their wishes and appoint someone to make decisions on their behalf if they become unable to do so.

Advanced directives are legal documents that outline a person's preferences for medical care in the event that they are unable to make decisions for themselves. This can include a living will, which outlines a person's wishes for end-of-life care, and a durable power of attorney for healthcare, which designates a person to make medical decisions on behalf of the individual. In hospice care, it is important for patients and their families to have advanced directives in place to ensure that the patient's end-of-life wishes are respected and followed.

The hospice case manager plays a key role in helping patients and their families to understand the importance of advanced directives and to complete the necessary documentation. This may involve discussing the different options available and helping the patient and their family to make informed decisions about their care. It may also involve assisting with the completion of the necessary paperwork and ensuring that it is properly filed and made available to the appropriate healthcare providers.

Additionally, the hospice case manager has a responsibility to ensure that these documents are followed and respected. This may involve communicating the patient's wishes to other members of the hospice care team and advocating for the patient's rights and preferences to be honored. The hospice case manager should also be prepared to provide emotional and spiritual support to the patient and their family as they navigate the end-of-life process and make difficult decisions about their care.

It is not uncommon for families to disagree with a patient's advanced directives, especially if the patient's wishes differ from what the family would prefer. In these situations, it can be challenging for the hospice case manager to navigate the conflicting desires of the patient and their family. It is important for the hospice case manager to be a neutral party in these situations and to respect the wishes of the patient, as long as they have the capacity to make their own decisions. The hospice case manager can work with the patient and their family to facilitate open and honest communication, and to help everyone understand the patient's goals for their care.

The hospice case manager can also help the patient and their family explore their options and come to a resolution that is in the best interests of the patient. In cases where the patient lacks the capacity to make their own decisions, the hospice case manager should work with the patient's power of attorney or legal guardian to ensure that the patient's wishes are respected to the greatest extent possible.

Power of attorney (POA) refers to a legal document that gives someone else the authority to make decisions on your behalf. This person is known as the attorney-in-fact or agent. There are several different types of POA, including general POA, durable POA, and medical POA.

General POA grants the attorney-in-fact broad powers to handle the principal's financial and legal affairs. Durable POA remains in effect even if the principal becomes incapacitated or unable to make decisions for themselves. Medical POA specifically gives the attorney-in-fact the authority to make healthcare decisions on behalf of the principal.

Medical power of attorney, also known as a healthcare power of attorney, is a legal document that allows someone to appoint another person to make healthcare decisions on their behalf if they are unable to do so. This person is known as the healthcare agent or surrogate decision-maker. The purpose of medical power of attorney is to ensure that the person's healthcare wishes are respected, even if they are unable to speak for themselves.

Medical power of attorney is an important aspect of end-of-life planning and is often included in a comprehensive advance directive. It is important for individuals to think about and discuss their healthcare preferences with their family and healthcare provider and to appoint a healthcare agent whom they trust to carry out their wishes.

In the hospice setting, the hospice case manager may be involved in discussing medical power of attorney with the patient and their family. It is important for the case manager to understand the patient's wishes and to help facilitate communication between the patient, their family, and the healthcare team. The case manager may also help the patient and their family understand the legal implications of medical power of attorney and ensure that the necessary documents are in place.

The durable POA is an important tool in hospice care, as it allows the patient to appoint someone they trust to make decisions on their behalf if they become unable to do so due to their illness. The durable POA can be used to make financial decisions, healthcare decisions, or both, depending on the specific terms of the document. The hospice case manager can play a role in helping the patient and their family understand the importance of having a durable POA in place and can assist in the process of creating and executing the document.

It is important to note that the durable POA is only effective if it is properly executed and meets the legal requirements of the state in which it is created. The hospice case manager can help ensure that the durable POA is properly prepared and executed to avoid any potential issues or disputes in the future.

It is important for individuals to consider their end-of-life wishes and to consider appointing a POA to ensure that their wishes are carried out. In the context of hospice care, the POA may be involved in making decisions related to the patient's care and treatment. The hospice case manager should work with the patient and their POA to ensure that the patient's wishes are respected and that the POA is able to make informed decisions on behalf of the patient.

Another key component of advanced care planning is making decisions about life-sustaining treatments. These are medical treatments that are designed to prolong life but may also cause discomfort or suffering. Examples of life-sustaining treatments include mechanical ventilation, dialysis, and artificial nutrition and hydration.

When making decisions about life-sustaining treatments, it is important to consider the potential benefits and risks of each treatment. This may involve discussing patients' preferences and values, as well as their prognosis and overall health. It may also involve consulting with other members of the healthcare team, such as doctors and chaplains, to provide comprehensive guidance.

A *Do Not Resuscitate (DNR)* order is a medical directive that instructs healthcare providers not to perform cardiopulmonary resuscitation (CPR) in the event that a patient's heart stops or they stop breathing. These orders are typically used by patients who have terminal illnesses or other conditions that make CPR unlikely to be successful.

In the hospice setting, a DNR order is often discussed with the patient and their family as part of the end-of-life planning process. The hospice case manager can help facilitate this conversation and provide information about the potential benefits and drawbacks of a DNR order. For example, a DNR order can help ensure that a patient is not subjected to unnecessary or unwanted medical interventions at the end of life, but it can also raise ethical and legal issues if the patient or their family disagrees with the decision.

It is important for the hospice case manager to respect the patient's autonomy and decision-making capacity when discussing a DNR order. The case manager should also ensure that the patient's wishes are clearly documented and communicated to the healthcare team and any other relevant parties. In some cases, a DNR order may need to be revisited or modified as the patient's condition changes. The hospice case manager should be prepared to facilitate these discussions and support the patient and their family through the decision-making process.

In addition to discussing end-of-life wishes and making decisions about life-sustaining treatments, advanced care planning also involves providing bereavement support to families after a patient's death. This may include providing emotional and practical support, such as helping with funeral arrangements and providing referrals to grief counseling.

When providing bereavement support, it is important to be sensitive to the unique needs and circumstances of each family. This may involve providing emotional support, such as listening and providing a supportive presence, as well as practical support, such as helping with funeral arrangements and providing referrals to grief counseling. It may also involve working with other members of the healthcare team, such as chaplains and social workers, to provide comprehensive support.

In addition to providing support for emotional and practical needs, it is also important for hospice case managers to provide support for spiritual and religious needs. Many families may have strong spiritual or religious beliefs and may want to incorporate these into their bereavement and end-of-life planning. As a hospice case manager, you may need to work with chaplains or other spiritual leaders to provide support in this area.

Advanced care planning is an important part of the work of the hospice case manager. By discussing patients' end-of-life wishes, making decisions about life-sustaining treatments, and providing bereavement support, the hospice case manager can help patients and their families to make informed decisions about their care, and to ensure that their wishes are respected and carried out.

Chapter 10

Hospice Care and the Important Role of the Case Manager

Hospice care is a specialized form of healthcare that focuses on providing comfort and support to patients who are facing a terminal illness or approaching the end of their lives. It is designed to help patients and their families manage the physical, emotional, and spiritual challenges that come with a terminal diagnosis and to provide support and comfort throughout the end-of-life journey. The positive impact of hospice care on patients and their families is immeasurable. By focusing on comfort and quality of life, hospice care helps patients, and their families make the most of the time they have left together.

The importance of the hospice case manager in providing high-quality care cannot be overstated. The hospice case manager is responsible for coordinating care and communication with the patient, their family, and other members of the hospice care team. They are also responsible for ensuring that the patient's care plan is being followed and that their goals and wishes are being respected. The hospice case manager plays a vital role in providing symptom management and emotional support to the patient and their family, as well as helping them navigate the complex healthcare system and make decisions about end-of-life care.

Being a hospice nurse case manager can be a rewarding but challenging role. One of the main challenges is the emotional toll of working with terminally ill patients and their families. It can be difficult to witness patients suffering and to provide support to families as they grieve the loss of a loved one. Another challenge is coordinating care with a multidisciplinary team, including physicians, nurses, chaplains, social workers, and volunteers. The hospice case manager must be organized and able to effectively communicate with all members of the team to ensure that the patient's care is consistent and aligned with their goals.

Despite these challenges, the role of the hospice case manager is crucial in providing compassionate, high-quality care to terminally ill patients and their families. Hospice care is a vital service that helps patients, and their families make the most of the time they have left together, and it provides a sense of peace and closure as they near the end of life. Being a hospice case manager is an incredibly rewarding career. It requires a deep understanding of end-of-life care and the ability to connect with patients and their families in a meaningful way.

Those who choose to become hospice case managers can make a positive difference in the lives of patients and their families during one of the most difficult times in their lives. They also have the opportunity to connect with an amazing community of healthcare professionals who are working together to provide comfort and care to those who are facing the end of their lives. They are an important part of the hospice team who provide the support and care for terminally ill patients and their families.

The hospice case manager plays an important role in educating patients and their families about hospice care. This includes educating them about the different levels of care available, the services offered by the hospice team, and what to expect during the end-of-life process. The hospice case manager should also be able to provide information about advanced care planning and end-of-life decision-making, as well as resources for bereavement support.

As the primary caregiver for patients and their families, the hospice case manager must also be able to provide emotional support and guidance. This includes being able to listen to patients and their families, validate their feelings, and provide a safe space for them to express their emotions. The hospice case manager must also be able to provide support and guidance to patients and their families as they navigate the end-of-life process, including dealing with grief and loss.

The role of the hospice case manager includes being an advocate for patients and their families. They must be able to communicate with other members of the healthcare team and ensure that the patient's goals and wishes are being respected. They must also be able to advocate for the patient's rights and ensure that they are receiving the appropriate level of care.

The hospice case manager plays an important role in the community. They can educate the community about the benefits of hospice care and the services offered by the hospice team. They can also assist families and caregivers in finding resources and support groups within the community. They can also help to increase awareness about end-of-life care, and advocate for policies and legislation that support hospice and palliative care. By building relationships and partnerships with other community organizations and healthcare providers, the hospice case manager can help to improve access to hospice care and support for patients and their families.

The hospice case manager must always be aware of the cultural and spiritual needs of patients and their families. They must be able to provide support and guidance that is sensitive to the patient's cultural and spiritual beliefs. This includes understanding and respecting the patient's beliefs about death and dying and providing appropriate bereavement support.

The hospice case manager must be aware of the changing healthcare landscape and stay informed of new developments and advancements in hospice care. This includes staying current with the latest research and best practices in hospice care, as well as new laws and regulations that may impact hospice care.

The hospice case manager must be able to work independently and as part of a team. They must be able to manage their time effectively, prioritize tasks, and meet deadlines. They must also be able to work collaboratively with other members of the hospice team to provide the best possible care for patients and their families.

The hospice case manager must be committed to their own personal and professional growth. This includes continuing their education, seeking out opportunities for professional development, and staying up to date with the latest developments in hospice care. They must also be committed to self-care, as the emotional demands of working with terminally ill patients and their families can take a toll on one's well-being. Regularly engaging in self-care activities such as exercise, mindfulness practices, and social support can help the hospice case manager to manage stress and maintain a healthy work-life balance. Additionally, they should also be open to seeking professional counseling or other mental health support as needed. Being self-aware and taking proactive steps to maintain their own well-being is essential to providing the best possible care to patients and their families.

Another important aspect of the hospice case manager's role is working with patients and their families to help them make informed decisions about their care. This may involve discussing end-of-life wishes, making decisions about life-sustaining treatments, and providing bereavement support after a patient's death. The hospice case manager must have the knowledge and skills necessary to help patients and their families understand the options available to them and make decisions that align with their values and beliefs.

It is important for the hospice case manager to be able to provide support to patients and their families in a variety of settings. This includes providing care in patients' homes, in long-term care facilities, and in hospice inpatient centers. The hospice case manager must be able to adapt to different environments and provide the appropriate level of care in each setting.

The hospice case manager also plays an important role in the continuity of care for patients and their families. This includes ensuring that patients receive the appropriate level of care as their condition changes, and that their care plan is updated accordingly. It also includes ensuring that patients and their families are provided with appropriate follow-up care and support after the patient's death.

The hospice case manager plays an important role in the quality improvement process of hospice care. They must be able to identify areas of improvement, develop and implement plans to address these areas, and measure the effectiveness of these plans. They must also be able to communicate with other members of the hospice care team and report on the progress of quality improvement initiatives. This ensures that the hospice care provided to patients and their families is of the highest quality and meets the standards set by regulatory bodies.

In conclusion, hospice care is a specialized form of healthcare that focuses on providing comfort and support to patients who are facing a terminal illness or approaching the end of their lives. The role of the hospice case manager is crucial in providing high-quality care to patients and their families during this difficult time. The hospice case manager is responsible for coordinating care, communicating with the patient and their family, and ensuring that the patient's care plan is being followed.

In summary, hospice care is a vital service that helps patients and their families make the most of the time they have left together. The role of the hospice case manager is essential in providing compassionate, high-quality care to patients and their families during the end-of-life process. The hospice case manager plays a vital role in providing support and guidance to patients and their families, and in ensuring that patients receive the appropriate level of care. The hospice case manager plays an important role in the continuity of care, in the quality improvement process, and in the community. They provide a vital service and make a positive difference in the lives of patients and their families during difficult times.

Dear fellow Hospice RN Case Manager,

I want to dedicate this space to expressing my heartfelt gratitude for the incredible work that you do every day. As hospice nurses, we have the unique and special privilege of serving patients and families during a very challenging and often emotionally difficult time in their lives. The care and compassion that you bring to your work is truly inspiring, and it is a true joy to witness the positive impact that you have on the lives of those in your care.

Your role as a hospice nurse is so multifaceted and vital in improving the quality of life for patients facing the end of their lives and their families. Whether it is through providing physical comfort through medication management and symptom control, offering emotional support and guidance to both patients and their loved ones, or simply being present and lending a listening ear, you make a tremendous difference in the lives of your patients. Your dedication to your patients and their families is truly admirable, and I am grateful to have the opportunity to work alongside such compassionate and caring colleagues.

I also wanted to congratulate you on choosing such an amazing and rewarding career. Being a hospice nurse requires a special kind of strength, compassion, and dedication, and I am so proud to be a part of this special community of healthcare professionals. It is a privilege to be able to serve others in this way, and I am grateful to have the opportunity to work alongside such dedicated and compassionate colleagues like you.

I hope that you will continue to find joy and fulfillment in your work, and please know that your hard work and dedication are deeply appreciated. You are making a difference in the lives of so many people, and your efforts are truly valued and admired. Please do not hesitate to reach out to me for support or encouragement as we navigate this challenging but deeply rewarding profession together.

Sincerely,

Frank M. Owen II, BSN, RN

Glossary

Activities of Daily Living (ADLs) *(Chapter 4)* - basic tasks of everyday life, such as bathing, dressing, and using the toilet, that are necessary for a person to live independently

Advanced directives *(Chapter 9)* - written instructions outlining a person's preferences for medical treatment in the event that they are unable to make decisions for themselves

CAUTI *(Chapter 4)* - Catheter-Associated Urinary Tract Infection, an infection of the urinary tract that occurs when a catheter

Certificate of Terminal Illness *(Chapter 1)* - a document stating that a patient has a terminal illness and has a life expectancy of six months or less

Comfort Kit *(Chapter 4)* - a kit of medications provided to hospice patients to help them manage symptoms and improve their comfort

Contractures *(Chapter 4)* - a tightening of the muscles or tendons around a joint that can lead to stiffness and difficulty moving

Consent for treatment form *(Chapter 7)* - a document in which a patient gives consent for a specific treatment or procedure

Death rattle *(Chapter 4)* - a sound that may occur when a person is near death due to secretions in the throat

Death visit *(Chapter 6)* - a visit by a hospice team to a patient who is expected to die within a short time frame

Dementia *(Chapter 8)* - a decline in cognitive function, including memory, language, and problem-solving abilities

Do Not Resuscitate (DNR) *(Chapter 9)* - a medical order stating that a person should not be resuscitated if their heart stops or they stop breathing

Durable Medical Equipment (DME) *(Chapter 4)* - medical equipment that is used for a long period of time and is intended to help a person maintain their independence

FAST scale *(Chapter 1)* - a tool used to assess for changes in mental status in patients with dementia

Fluid overload *(Chapter 4)* - excess of fluid in the body

General Inpatient or GIP *(Chapter 5)* - a level of hospice care in which the patient receives inpatient care for pain or symptom management that cannot be managed in other settings

Hospice *(Chapter 1)* - a type of healthcare that focuses on providing comfort and support to patients and their families during the end-of-life process

Hospice election form *(Chapter 7)* - a document in which a patient elects to receive hospice care

In-service *(Chapter 5)* - a training session provided by a professional to educate and update the knowledge and skills of family members or facility staff on a specific topic related to their field of work

Informed consent *(Chapter 7)* - a process in which a patient is provided with information about a treatment or procedure and gives their consent for it to be performed

Interdisciplinary team (IDT) or interdisciplinary group (IDG) meeting *(Chapter 1)* - a meeting of the hospice team to discuss and coordinate the patient's care

Kennedy terminal ulcer *(Chapter 4)* - a type of pressure wound that occurs on the lower legs of patients with advanced terminal illnesses

Medicare Hospice Benefit *(Chapter 1)* - a Medicare benefit that provides hospice care to people with a terminal illness

National Hospice and Palliative Care Organization (NHPCO) *(Chapter 1)* - a professional association for hospice and palliative care providers

Non-pharmacologic pain control *(Chapter 4)* - refers to the use of methods other than medication to manage and relieve pain

Nursing diagnosis *(Chapter 3)* - a clinical judgment about an individual, family, or community response to actual or potential health problems/life processes

Palliative care *(Chapter 9)* - medical care that focuses on providing relief from the symptoms, pain, and stress of a serious illness

PAINAD *(Chapter 8)* - a tool used to assess pain in patients who are unable to communicate their pain verbally

Power of Attorney *(Chapter 9)* - a legal document in which a person gives someone else the authority to make decisions on their behalf

PPS scale *(Chapter 1)* - a tool used to assess the functional status of patients in hospice care

Pressure wounds (pressure ulcers / bedsores) *(Chapter 4)* - wounds that occur when constant pressure on the skin cuts off blood flow and damages skin and underlying tissue

Recertification visit *(Chapter 1)* - a visit by a hospice team to determine whether the patient continues to meet the criteria for hospice care

Rally *(Chapter 6)* - a temporary improvement in a patient's condition after a period of decline

Silver Tsunami *(Chapter 8)* - a term used to describe the aging of the population and the resulting increase in the number of older adults

Stages of death *(Chapter 6)* - the final stages of life leading up to death, including the pre-active, active, and dying stages

Terminal diagnosis *(Chapter 1)* - a diagnosis stating that a patient has a terminal illness and has a life expectancy of six months or less

Terminal fever *(Chapter 4)* - a sudden and persistent rise in body temperature that may occur in the final stages of life

Made in the USA
Monee, IL
12 May 2023

6f4f3b98-2dfc-4e67-8e1a-611bbf725555R02